D0830038

DISCARD

KINKY COILY

A Natural Hair Resource Guide

PAMELA SAMUELS YOUNG

KINKY COILY

A Natural Hair Resource Guide

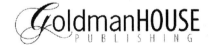

Kinky Coily: A Natural Hair Resource Guide

Goldman House Publishing
ISBN 978-0-9857341-6-9
First Edition
Copyright © 2014 by Pamela Samuels Young

All rights reserved. No part of this book may be reproduced, transmitted or used in whole or in part in any form by any electronic, mechanical or other means now known or hereafter invented, including, but not limited to, xerography, photocopying and recording, or by any information storage or retrieval system, without the express written permission of Goldman House Publishing. The only exception shall be in the case of short quotations embodied in a review, article or other non-commercial use permitted by copyright laws. The products, brands and company names used in this book are referenced only for proper identification without the intent to infringe or violate the rights of any trademark holder. For information about special discounts for bulk purchases, please contact the author or Goldman House Publishing.

Pamela Samuels Young
AuthorPamelaSamuelsYoung@gmail.com

Goldman House Publishing
GoldmanHousePublishing@gmail.com

Cover design by Marion Designs

Printed in U.S.A.

R0444386531

BOOKS BY
PAMELA SAMUELS YOUNG

Vernetta Henderson Mysteries

Every Reasonable Doubt (1st in series)

In Firm Pursuit (2nd in series)

Murder on the Down Low (3rd in series)

Attorney-Client Privilege (4th in series)

Angela Evans Mysteries

Buying Time (1st in series)

Anybody's Daughter (2nd in series)

Short Stories

The Setup

Easy Money

Non-Fiction

Kinky Coily: A Natural Hair Resource Guide

Kinky Coily Natural Hair Journal

DISCLAIMER

The reader should use his or her best judgment when utilizing the resources and information contained in this book. The author is not a hair care professional and her recommendations and advice are based primarily on her own hair care experiences. As such, the information, resources, products, and individuals referenced in this book are provided for general informational purposes only, and should not be used or relied upon for any diagnostic or treatment purposes.

While the author and publisher strive to make the information contained herein as timely and as accurate as possible, they make no promises, guarantees or representations of any kind, express or implied, about the reliability, adequacy, completeness, accuracy, or suitability of the information in this book, and expressly disclaim liability for any errors or omissions contained herein. Any reliance placed upon the information contained in this book is taken strictly at your own risk. You are advised to consult with a hair care professional and/or a physician before using any of the products, information, resources or treatment methods referenced herein.

In no event shall the author or publisher be liable for any loss or damage alleged to be directly or indirectly caused by the advice, information, individuals or resources contained in this book, including without limitation, indirect, special, incidental, punitive or consequential damages of any kind, whether arising under breach of contract, tort (including negligence) strict liability or any other legal theory.

ACKNOWLEDGEMENTS

I'd like to thank those natural sisters and wannabe naturals who critiqued the manuscript for *Kinky Coily: A Natural Hair Resource Guide* and gave me much-needed feedback: Dr. Carline Louis-Jacques, Latrice Byrdsong, Akua Searcy, Arlene Walker, Robin Smith, Lessie Adams, Tammy Griffin, Judy Brown, Saba McKinley, Sharlene Moore, Kelly-Ann Henry and Linette Samuels.

To my assistant Lynel Washington, thanks for all you do! To the baddest publicist I know, Ella Curry of EDC Creations, thanks so much for spreading the word about this book! Now, Ella, if I could only get *you* back on your natural hair journey. That would indeed be an accomplishment!

DEDICATION

To Deanie Brewer and Alisa Covington,
Thanks for taking me on a natural hair journey and
leading me to the discovery of my fabulously kinky coils!

CONTENTS

Why I Wrote This Book

FIRST THINGS FIRST. I'M NOT a hair stylist or hair care professional. I've never gone to beauty school and I don't have a degree in anything even remotely related to hair care. So how in the heck do I have the audacity to write a book about natural hair? Well, in the midst of a desperate search for solutions to my own hair woes, I discovered a wealth of information about natural hair care. I was shocked and amazed at all the things I *didn't* know about the care and versatility of my own hair. I was even more shocked when I realized that many, if not most, hair stylists who care for kinky-textured hair don't know much about the true capabilities of our hair either. Why should they? The cosmetology schools certainly aren't teaching it. Once I had attained this priceless information, I was bursting at the seams to spread the gospel. I wasn't just content to share my knowledge with family, friends and strangers I met on the street. Since I'm a writer by trade, I decided to write the kind of book I desperately needed at the start of my journey: one that would point me in the direction of resources that would equip me with the necessary knowledge to care for my own hair.

Unfortunately, I've had a love-hate relationship with my hair for most of my life. It never grew as long as I wanted it to be (shoulder length). It wasn't as thick as I wanted it to be. Whether pressed or relaxed, it never stayed beauty-shop straight for more than a couple of days after leaving my stylist's chair. I'm happy to announce, however, that my days of complaining about my hair are over. Having discovered that I have naturally curly hair (who knew?), I'm now in the midst of a straight-up love affair with my tresses! My only regret is that I didn't come to appreciate the versatility of my wonderfully kinky coils years ago. I could have saved myself tons of time, money and hair drama.

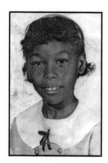 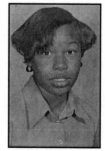

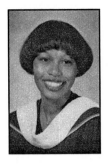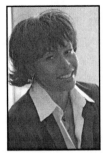

No one, certainly not me, could have ever predicted that *I* would become a YouTube blogger or write a book about natural hair. But after watching my relaxed hair shed excessively for weeks, I decided to take charge of my own hair care. My true natural hair care education developed in fits and starts. A YouTube video here, an Internet article there, a tip or product recommendation shared by a friend at a party or a stranger in the grocery store. With each bit of knowledge I attained, I continued to dig deeper. And deeper. And even deeper. I now consider myself a bona fide natural hair enthusiast and I'm passionate about sharing my newfound knowledge with the world.

I can still recall the precise moment that I decided to write this book. I was at Los Angeles International Airport headed out of town for a book signing for one of my mystery novels. I'd just finished making my way through the security checkpoint and was struggling to slip back into my shoes while simultaneously trying to retrieve my belongings from the gray plastic bucket on the conveyor belt. I had just grabbed my purse and laptop when I turned around and found myself face-to-face with an older female security agent.

"Ma'am, can you step this way?"

Dang!

I was running late and didn't have time for a pat down or a second scan of my carry-on bags. I hadn't had my morning coffee yet and if I didn't get going, I'd have to board my flight without a much-needed caffeine boost.

I grudgingly followed the agent a few feet away from the security check line. To my surprise, she didn't commence an immediate pat down. Instead, she leaned forward and whispered into my ear.

"Your hair is really cute. What did you do to get it like that?"

Relieved that I didn't have to go through any additional security-check hassles, I thanked her for the compliment, then gladly rattled off a couple of my favorite hair care products, quickly explained how I shingle my hair (more on that later) and encouraged her to give it a try. I then hurried off to find my departure gate and, hopefully, a Starbucks somewhere in the vicinity.

I quickly found both the gate and Starbucks. As luck would have it, the line was way longer than I needed it to be. I stepped in line anyway, checking my watch every few seconds hoping I could get my coffee before boarding commenced. When I finally made it up to the counter, the twenty-something barista scribbled my order on the side of a cup, but wasn't quite ready to close the transaction.

"How did you get your hair like that?" she asked.

For the second time that morning, I spouted off the products and technique I used to define my curls. This time (to the dismay of those in line behind me) I actually grabbed one of my curls and demonstrated the shingle technique.

"You should give it a try," I urged her. *Now can you put my order through?*

Coffee finally in hand, I took a seat near my gate with five precious minutes to spare before boarding began.

A woman sitting in the chair next to me pointed at my head.

"Your hair is so cute. I could never get *my* hair to look like that."

"Yes, you could." I eyed her short, pressed hair, whose texture appeared to be similar to mine. "Kinky hair has a natural curl pattern. You just need to find the right products."

"No way," she said, defiantly shaking her head.

For the third time that morning, I went through my spiel. This woman, however, wasn't buying it.

"I'd love to go natural," she said, her voice wistful. "But my hair is *way* too nappy to do anything with."

"Nappy hair is curly hair," I explained.

Her face scrunched up as if she'd suddenly realized that I might not be playing with a full deck.

"Uh…yeah, okay. If you say so."

As I was boarding the plane, I found myself wishing I'd had more time to convince this stranger that her *kinky* hair was actually *curly*. The most disheartening part of my natural hair journey was recognizing that most African-American women don't understand or appreciate the true texture of their hair. Before commencing my journey, I certainly didn't. I viewed my hair in its natural state as nappy, unruly and unworthy of ever being on public display. I had absolutely no idea that I had a natural curl pattern that could be defined with the right products.

As I settled in for takeoff, I started thinking about each of the women who'd approached me that morning. In less than twenty minutes, I'd come across three women—one older, one younger, and one close to me in age—who had no appreciation for all that their natural hair could be. I knew that there were thousands of other kinky-haired women in the same boat. After all, I used to be one of them. I promised myself that I would start carrying a sample of my favorite gel and the next time I met a stranger who insisted that her kinky hair was not naturally curly, I'd march her to the nearest bathroom, put her in front of a mirror and show her otherwise.

Then it hit me. *Why not write a book that exposed this hidden truth to all of my kinky-haired sisters?* I could share the natural hair resources that led me to open my eyes about my own hair and help other women see the true beauty of their textured tresses.

So here it is!

Whether you're simply thinking about starting a natural hair journey, just getting started or a natural hair pro, *Kinky Coily: A Natural Hair Resource Guide* has something for you.

CHAPTER 1

My Personal Journey to Natural Hair

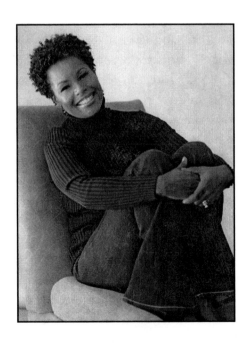

M E GO NATURAL? I DON'T think so!

For most of my life, I did not like my hair. Hence, the thought of going natural wasn't for me. I had lots of weak excuses for never even considering it.

My hair is too nappy.

My hair is too thin.

My forehead is too big.

I don't have the face for it.

It's not corporate.

Meanwhile, I tried it all: flat-ironing, relaxers, texturizers, weaves, extensions, micro-braids and cornrows. During all of those stages, I had no idea that I was trapped in a vicious cycle of growth and breakage. A couple of times in my life, my hair grew as long as the nape of my neck, but unfortunately it never stayed that way for long. In a matter of months, it had somehow broken off. Even though I was consistently under the care of a hair stylist, I could never retain any length. I just assumed that kinky hair—and my hair in particular—could not grow long.

My transition to natural hair and the discovery of the true magnificence of my kinky coils happened totally by accident. Actually, by *catastrophe* might be a more accurate description.

Oddly enough, during the period immediately prior to my transition, I was in the midst of a rather satisfying period with my hair. I was wearing it relaxer-free and flat-ironed, which I maintained with weekly visits to my hair stylist. Before that, I had been rocking micro braids for three years, having worn a relaxer then a weave prior to that. I loved my braids and the freedom of not having to hassle with styling my hair every day. I also experienced tremendous growth during the three-year period that I wore braids.

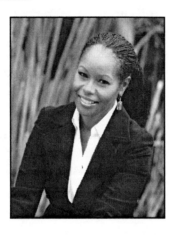

Now, for the first time since a short period in college, my hair was healthy and approaching shoulder length again.

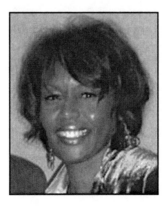

I was thrilled. Life was good.

But while I loved my flat-ironed hair, maintaining it was a big-time hassle. I couldn't work out with the vigor that I wanted because I didn't want to sweat my hair back to its natural state. Taking a shower required wrapping my head up like a mummy. Don't mention getting caught in the rain. And those dreaded hot flashes just made maintaining straight hair without a relaxer a completely futile effort. Finding the time in my crazy schedule to get to the beauty shop and the long commute to get there (nearly an hour one-way) was also getting old.

As I began to travel more frequently for book signings as well as my work as an in-house lawyer for a major corporation, I wanted my hair fresh when I hit the road. My stylist at the time taught me how to straighten my own hair and equipped me with a flat iron that used less heat. Once I realized I could wash and straighten my own hair, I was thrilled.

Still, there was the problem of my hair turning into a fro after a workout, shower or rainstorm. So I decided that returning to a relaxer would solve all of my problems.

Contrary to my stylist's directions, I began to use my flat iron between beauty shop visits way more than I should have. I absolutely loved the bounce and shine of my straightened hair right after washing, blow drying and flat ironing it.

I soon began to notice a sprinkling of short hairs in the sink every time I combed my hair. At first, it didn't bother me much. Hair is supposed to shed, right? By this time, I was doing my own hair once or twice a week and seeing my hair stylist every two to three weeks. And on top of that, I would often touch up my hair with the flat iron in between washes a couple times a week. What I didn't know then, but realize now is that the excessive heat from the blow drying, flat-ironing and heat styling was severely damaging my hair.

Since the breakage didn't happen all at once, I didn't recognize how excessive it was until most of the damage was done. Now, when I styled my hair in the morning, my sink wasn't just dotted with tiny hairs, it was *covered* with them! My shiny, bouncy hair no longer looked thick and full. It looked thin and scraggily. My edges— which had always been thin—were now nearly bald. At the back of my head, where I attached a fake ponytail with a built-in comb when I didn't feel like curling my hair, a big bald spot began to emerge. If you don't believe me, take a look at the pictures on the next page, which were taken after the damage was done.

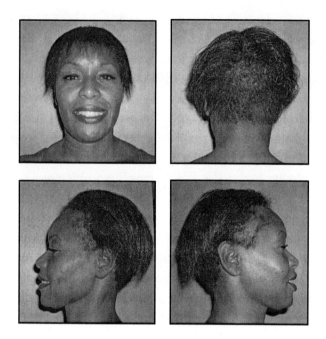

What in the heck was going on?

On my next beauty shop visit, I pointed out the bald spot to my stylist. She gave me a deep conditioner and measured the spot so that on my next visit, she could see if it was expanding. She advised me to stop using the flat iron and to get rid of my fake ponytail since it was the likely culprit for my alarming bald spot. Unfortunately, I didn't follow her advice about tossing the ponytail. Why? Because I had no other way to style my hair since it was now too short and thin to curl.

On my next visit a couple of weeks later, my hair stylist measured the bald patch at the back of my head again and confirmed that it *was* expanding. She again advised me to stop wearing the fake ponytail and gave me another deep conditioning treatment. By this time, I was done with the relaxer. I was determined to grow it out and never relax my hair again.

As I waited (quite impatiently) for my relaxer to grow out, the breakage and shedding continued at an alarming rate. Thank God for an outing with five of my closest girlfriends. *That evening altered my hair life forever.*

We'd gathered for dinner at a posh L.A. restaurant on Melrose Boulevard. I immediately noticed my friend Alisa's hair. It was thick and full—much thicker and fuller than the last time I remembered it.

When I complimented her hair, Alisa nonchalantly explained that she was "on a hair journey."

Huh?

"What's a hair journey?" I asked.

She waved me off, stating that it was too complicated to explain over dinner. She promised to send me an email telling me all about it the next day.

All through dinner, as we talked and gossiped, my mind was on Alisa's hair. Had she found some superstar hair stylist? My hair was falling out in gobs. I couldn't wait until tomorrow. I needed to know her secret now!

As we were leaving the restaurant, I reminded Alisa about her promise to follow up with me about her *hair journey.*

That night, Alisa forwarded a series of emails she had received from another friend of hers, Deanie. The emails contained links to YouTube videos of women— black women—who were blogging about their hair and teaching other women how to care for their own hair. I can still remember watching the *hair journey* videos posted on YouTube by bloggers Hairlista and Nunaavane. These sisters were not natural. They were pressed and permed with hair down their backs!

How could these women grow such long, healthy hair on their own without the aid of a hair stylist? Was this for real? The before and after pictures of their hair growth convinced me that it was.

I was totally mesmerized by the videos of my African-American and Caribbean sisters who were taking charge of their own hair care. What I saw left me in awe. I, like many people, assumed that *our* hair couldn't grow that long. The fact that they were growing their own healthy hair without the help of a hair stylist was nothing short of eye-opening. It also got me to thinking. Maybe *I* could resolve my own hair problems.

The day after my girls' night out, I checked into a hotel for some hibernation time to work on my next novel. But instead of writing, I spent *the entire time* on my laptop, devouring hair tips from YouTube bloggers. These videos empowered me. If these women could grow their own healthy hair, perhaps I could too. I canceled my hair appointment for the following week and started taking notes. I decided that I would take charge of my own hair care.

Later that day, Alisa drove almost an hour to my hotel to give me a bottle of Jamaican Black Castor Oil and gave me instructions on how to use it on my hair.

She also put me in touch with her friend Deanie. I later came to learn that Deanie was responsible for many, many women starting their own hair journeys.

In a fit of panic, I called Deanie and recounted my tragic hair loss woes. Although Deanie has never spent a day in beauty school and has never held a job in the hair care industry, she immediately took charge.

"First, we have to stop your hair breakage," Deanie declared over the phone, never having seen my hair.

She calmed me down and assured me that she *could* and *would* stop my hair loss. I'm not sure I really believed her, but I was so desperate I was willing to try anything.

Deanie graciously agreed to meet me at a beauty supply store near her home. We met up in the parking lot before going inside. I climbed into her car, pulled off my scarf and showed her my frayed hair, thinning edges and the expanding bald spot at the back of my head. She fingered my hair and immediately told me that my hair was dry and needed moisture. She also said a protein treatment would help. I followed her into the beauty supply store where she examined labels and picked out a series of products: a shampoo, a couple of deep conditioners, a protein treatment, moisturizers and oils.

She gave me instructions in a language that sounded foreign at the time: co-wash, pre-poo, sulfate-free. I took it all in and prayed that all this crazy talk would stop my hair from falling out. Deanie emailed me specific directions about how to use each product I'd purchased and in which order. She promised me that her concoctions would put an end to my hair breakage and sent me on my way.

Again, I wasn't one hundred percent sure that what she was telling me would work. But I did what she recommended because I had no other options.

I rushed back to the hotel and put what I've dubbed *The Deanie Treatment* to work.

I didn't know it at the time, but Deanie was recommending the tips that the natural hair bloggers on YouTube have been publicizing to the world for years:

1. co-washing or using a sulfate-free shampoo;
2. weekly deep conditioning;
3. daily moisturizing and sealing;
4. regular protein treatments;
5. avoidance of heat; and
6. protective styling.

Something miraculous happened after I followed Deanie's directions. *My hair breakage stopped. Immediately.* The next morning as I combed through my hair, I was amazed. The sink was no longer covered with tiny broken hairs as had been the case *every day* for the past several weeks. *After applying that first deep conditioning treatment that Deanie recommended, I have never again experienced that kind of excessive breakage and shedding.*

Okay, so *now* I'm a true believer.

I didn't write a word of my novel that weekend. I continued watching YouTube videos and taking notes about what was good and bad for my hair. I made a list of products I wanted to try and created a weekly regimen for treating my damaged hair.

Deanie continued to send me emails and I soaked up her advice and supplemented it with what I was learning on my own. I threw out my sulfate-laden shampoo and started co-washing (using conditioner rather than shampoo to clean my hair). I put my flat iron and blow dryer on the shelf and moisturized and sealed my hair every night. I also deep conditioned one or two times a week.

Although the bloggers talked about the "big chop"—cutting off the relaxed or damaged hair and leaving just your natural hair texture—I couldn't bring myself to do anything that drastic. But I needed a protective style until my hair grew back. My friend Karen told me about a natural-looking wig one of her co-workers was wearing called the Mommy wig. The wig looked so natural, in fact, Karen thought it was her co-worker's real hair. When I searched for the wig on YouTube, up popped the talented blogger, Coloured Beautiful. As she demonstrated how to style the wig, I wondered if the Mommy wig would be a good look for me. It was. For the next

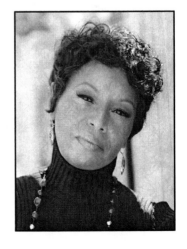

few months, I kept my thinning hair hidden underneath my very fashionable wig and prayed for it to grow.

Still, at this point in my hair journey, I had no plans to wear my hair *natural*. My only goal was to grow out my relaxer and return to wearing it in a flat-ironed style. The natural look just wasn't for me. Both Deanie and Alisa had beautiful straightened hair. My goal was to grow my hair thick and long like theirs.

After about four months, however, I got fed up with the wig and decided to take a very bold step—at least it was bold for me. I made up my mind to do the big chop and go natural!

Two things prompted that decision. First, I found wearing a wig to be a big-time hassle. The wig cap was irritating and I didn't like keeping my hair smothered all the time, especially as we entered the hot summer months. Second, and more importantly, by happenstance, I ran across a product review on YouTube by Coloured Beautiful. After seeing her Mommy wig video, I'd started checking out her YouTube videos on a regular basis and tried to master her fantastic makeup tips. But on this occasion, she was doing a product review of Kinky Curly Curling Custard. I watched as she applied the product to her natural hair and it transformed into *curly* hair. *Hmmmmm.* Would Kinky Curly Curling Custard do the same thing to *my* hair? I ran to my nearest Whole Foods and purchased a jar of the gel-like custard and applied it to my new growth. *OMG!*

Right before my eyes, my natural curl pattern emerged! (Check out my YouTube videos *How to Determine Your Curl Pattern* and *How to Get the Kinky Coily Look*. You'll find them on my YouTube channel Kinky Coily Pamela.)

For the record, nearly a year earlier, before I had a relaxer, I do recall my former hair stylist pointing out to me that I had a natural curl pattern. She had just finished washing my hair and after she applied conditioner, my hair waved up.

"You have a really nice curl pattern," she told me, showing me my curls over the shampoo bowl.

She then told me that I could wear my hair curly and recommended that I use the Mixed Chicks leave-in conditioner and said that would do the trick. The product did define my curls...but only until my hair dried. An hour later, my hair looked like a big fuzzy cotton ball. So after that, I abandoned the idea that I could wear my hair naturally curly. What I didn't understand at the time was that my particular hair texture needed a heavier product, like a gel, to keep my curls defined.

Okay, back to my story. Only after discovering that Kinky Curly Curling Custard defined my curls and kept them that way even *after* my hair had dried, did I have the confidence to do the big chop. I had a different hair stylist cut off all of my perm-damaged hair, leaving me with just a few inches of my naturally kinky hair.

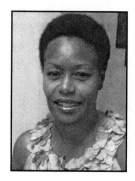 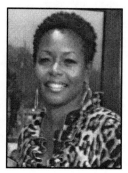

The big chop was both a frightening and liberating experience. But I'm happy to report that the hair drama I experienced (as evidenced by those pictures on page 12) is history.

One year after my big chop, I decided to straighten my hair for New Year's Eve. I wanted to compare the current state of my hair to the way it looked at the beginning of my journey when it was severely damaged and breaking off on a daily basis.

Take a look at my progress on the next page!

It was such an empowering experience to successfully manage my own hair care. Like many women with kinky hair, I was raised to believe that I was not equipped to care for my own hair. Only a licensed cosmetologist had the proper skills to manage my unruly textured tresses. I was wrong. Thanks to my YouTube sisters, I took the initiative and acquired the knowledge and skills to care for my own hair and you can too.

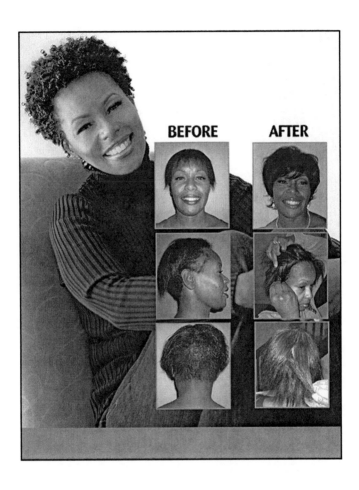

So are you a believer now? Then let's get started on *your* natural hair journey!

CHAPTER 2

Getting Started

A S YOU BEGIN YOUR NATURAL hair journey, you'll quickly find that there's a lot to learn. Have no fear. It can be done! The learning curve in terms of understanding the basics of natural hair care is not only fast, but fun. Once you discover the versatility and beauty of your natural hair, you'll wonder why you didn't go natural sooner. And before you know it, you'll be bringing other women into the fold.

At times, you may find this book and all that goes into going natural a bit overwhelming. Honestly, in the beginning of my journey, I certainly did. So I won't kid you. Going natural, particularly if you're transitioning from a relaxer or damaged hair, will take some work. But armed with your commitment and the resources provided in this book, your natural hair journey will be a resounding success.

Before we cover some of the basics of natural hair care, let's begin by defining a couple of terms you'll hear quite a bit on your journey: *natural hair* and *transitioning.*

What is Natural Hair?

Merriam-Webster's dictionary defines the word "natural" as *existing in nature and not made or caused by people; coming from nature.* Also: *not having any extra substances or chemicals added; not containing anything artificial.*

Wikipedia provides this definition of natural Afro-textured hair:

> *Afro-textured hair is a term used to refer to the natural texture of Black African hair that has not been altered by hot combs, flat irons, or chemicals (through perming, relaxing or straightening).*

I wanted to begin this section by defining "natural" to make the point that going natural may mean different things to different people. After being natural for about a year, I decided to flat-iron my hair for New Year's Eve. The intent was always to return to my kinky coils after the celebrating was over. I was curious to see how much my hair had progressed since going natural.

I was shocked at how many people let me know that I had committed some kind of sin by straightening my hair. Even when I wore micro braids as a protective style for a couple of months, a few people questioned my commitment to natural hair.

At the outset, I want to say that I personally define being natural as avoiding the use of chemicals which permanently alter the hair structure. For others, however, going natural means *never*, even temporarily, altering your hair structure. By that definition using a flat iron to straighten the hair is out. And there are still others who feel that using products such as gels to define your curls is not truly "natural".

As you begin your natural hair journey, you will run across all kinds of factions and debates on this topic. My advice? Go with the definition that works for you. One of the things I like most about my hair is its versatility. I can rock my hair kinky, straight or braided at the snap of a finger. And as far as I'm concerned, as long as I'm not putting a relaxer in my hair, I'm natural!

What is Transitioning?

If you have a chemical relaxer in your hair, transitioning is the process of allowing the relaxer to grow out until it's replaced with your new growth, *i.e.*, your natural, God-given hair texture. In my opinion—and maybe mine alone—transitioning is also moving away from the flat iron or straightening comb and wearing your hair in its natural state. Of course, transitioning from flat-ironed hair is a much easier process than transitioning from a relaxer.

I'll be completely honest with you. Transitioning can be a frustrating process. It was for me. It was frustrating primarily due to the slow growth of my hair. Every few weeks, I would clip the ends of my relaxed hair and check for new growth. Needless to say, my constant search for growth was a useless exercise. As my first hair mentor Deanie warned me, "A watched pot never boils."

Depending on your hair goals as well as the length and condition of your hair, transitioning can take months or years. That's why many women forgo the transitioning process and move straight to the big chop. How you decide to transition is completely up to you.

A Quick Preview

Here's a quick preview of what you'll learn in the following chapters of *Kinky Coily: A Natural Hair Resource Guide.*

In Chapter 3, *The Journey*, your natural hair education is divided into three easy steps.

STEP ONE
Master the Fundamentals of Natural Hair Care
In this section you'll be introduced to the basics of natural hair care, such as the lingo, the tools and products you'll need, the different hair textures and curl patterns, as well as techniques to care for your hair, which will likely be quite different from how you've been taught to care for your kinky coils.

STEP TWO
Create Your Natural Hair Go To Team
In the next section you'll learn where to find the best resources (bloggers, books, magazines, natural hair communities and more) for advice on growing and maintaining healthy natural hair. These resources will be instrumental in your journey. When you hit a roadblock, your Go To Team is where you will turn for help.

STEP THREE
Design Your Personal Natural Hair Care Regimen
The third section is where you'll create a hair care regimen that fits your specific needs. I've even included my own regimens as examples to help you get started.

In Chapter 4, *Relax and Enjoy the Journey!* that's exactly what you'll be instructed to do. You'll receive words of caution and encouragement as you begin your natural hair journey. At times, this motivation will be just what the doctor ordered.

Finally, in Chapter 5, *Resources*, I've shared some of my favorite natural hair care staples, such as recipes and products. I've also included an extensive list of books and bloggers as well as companies with natural hair product lines.

How to Use This Book

Kinky Coily: A Natural Hair Resource Guide is exactly that, *a resource guide.* All the answers to your natural hair care needs are not contained in these pages. You'll have to do more research on your own to truly reach a comfort level in caring for your natural hair. This book is simply a tool to get you started. Like any learning process, whether you achieve your goals will depend on how much effort you put into it. Here are a few tips that will hopefully help this book work for you.

Take Good Notes

As you're reading this book, make sure you have pen and paper handy so you can jot down notes as you read. Or you may prefer to take notes on your computer, laptop, tablet or smartphone. I've created a *Hair Care* file in the Notes app on my iPhone where I write down important hair care information, such as tips, recipes or products I want to try out. I also like to highlight helpful passages in books I read with a yellow highlighter. If you're reading this book on an e-reader, you can use your device's *highlight* and *notes* functions for this purpose.

If you're really serious about this journey (as I hope you are), I would strongly urge you to begin keeping a natural hair journal. You can use the tips in Chapter 3 to create your own journal or purchase the journal that accompanies this book, *The Kinky Coily Natural Hair Journal* (available at Amazon.com). My first natural hair journal was a monthly planner that I picked up at a stationery store. I chose one that had sufficient space for me to write down what treatments I used on a particular day, as well as space in the back to list products and make notes about things that worked well and those that didn't. You'll also want to record your overall thoughts about how your journey is progressing. I think it's important to use a calendar that allows you to see the month at a glance. That way, it's easy for you to quickly determine how long it's been between washes, deep conditioning, and other treatments.

Read, Then Watch

After reading the first two sections in Chapter 3 (*Step One–Master the Fundamentals of Natural Hair Care* and *Step Two–Build Your Natural Hair Care Go To Team*) I suggest that you set aside a few hours to watch several natural hair videos on YouTube before finishing the rest of the book.

I recommend that you begin by watching a few *journey* videos. These are videos where naturals document the progress of their hair journey with photographs. This will give you a big dose of motivation. Here are a few of my favorite journey videos on YouTube:

- Mahogany Curls, *Natural Hair Journey 2009-2011*

- Nikkimae2003, *Mae's 4 Year Natural Hair Journey*

- Kimmaytube, *LUVNaturals #17 My YouTube Hair Journey* (Parts 1 and 2).

Please be sure to also watch my YouTube channel, Kinky Coily Pamela, and my video, *My Transition to Natural Hair: The First 9 Months.*

Also, before continuing with the rest of the book, take some time to soak up some words of wisdom from a few of the true (in my opinion) natural hair experts on YouTube. My favorites include Curly Nikki, Urbanbushbabes, Mahogany Curls, Naptural85, and KimmayTube. (Also see the Natural Hair Bloggers on page 90 for more fabulous bloggers.) These sisters are incredibly knowledgeable about the care of kinky-textured hair. Just select a topic of interest to you and listen up. Two of the best websites on natural hair care (again, just my opinion) are CurlyNikki.com and BlackgirlLongHair.com. You should definitely browse those sites as well, before returning to this book.

A word of caution: natural hair blogs can be addictive! You may plan to spend an hour or so browsing YouTube, but look up and find that four or five hours have passed you by!

Four Natural Hair Must-Haves

I know, I know. You're super excited and anxious to get started on your natural hair journey. You've been admiring other naturals and you can't wait to rock your own kinky coils. Just hold on a minute.

Beginning a natural hair journey is going to require that you think differently about your hair. You will need to believe that *you* alone, if you so choose, can maintain your own hair. While the process will be frustrating at times, it will also be rewarding and empowering. If you make the commitment, I guarantee that you'll end up with an appreciation of your kinky coils and a greater confidence in yourself.

Here are four things you *must* possess in order to have a successful natural hair journey.

A New Mindset

It is essential that you embrace a whole new mindset about the beauty of your hair to make a successful transition to natural hair. Many of us with kinky hair have been raised to believe that we cannot take care of our own hair, that our hair is unruly, difficult and just plain "bad." That's bull.

I began getting my hair done at the beauty shop around the age of 12. Before that, my mother wrestled with me and a hot comb, occasionally leaving me with burn marks on my neck and ears. (Sorry, Mama, I know you tried!) My mother ultimately threw in the towel and handed me over to a neighborhood beautician. Over the next several years, I spent every other Saturday with Mrs. Meeks, who pressed me straight, greased up my scalp, and curled me up tighter than a water bug.

As I moved from city to city, the first thing I did after getting settled in (and sometimes before) was to find a hair stylist. Never once did it cross my mind that *I* could do my own hair.

Even after watching the first videos of those take-charge bloggers on YouTube, it took me a while to really *believe* that I could manage the care of my own hair. At the start of my journey, I had simply planned to grow out my relaxer and go back to flat-ironing my hair. The natural look was not for me. Why? Sadly, it's been en-grained in us that straight hair is good hair and kinky hair is bad. I admit it. I drank the Kool-Aid in gulps.

But my view and appreciation of my kinky hair slowly began to change. I am so pleased to now see an explosion of interest in natural hair, as evidenced by the expanding number of products, bloggers, websites, books and conferences dedicated to natural hair. When you see Oprah on the cover of *O* magazine with natu-ral hair (check out the September 2012 issue), you know something major is going on.

So I urge you to start your natural hair journey with an open mind. Allow your hair to be all that it can be and love it for its beauty and flexibility. How many non-kinky-haired women can sport straight hair, kinky curls, twists, buns, bantu knots, micro-braids *and* cornrows. None I know.

You're going to have to erase all those negative no-tions you have about what your hair can and cannot do. You have the most fabulous hair on the planet. Embrace it!

Time

I've heard many women say that going natural takes too much work. Really? I can remember spending three-to-four hours in the beauty shop, and that didn't include my nearly two-hour, round-trip commute. If I was getting a weave, the entire day and night might be lost.

Before you commit to making the transition to natural hair, I urge you to take a moment to consider how much time and effort you want to commit to this process. You may decide that it's way too much work for you and you'd prefer to hand over the reins to a natural hair stylist. That's a choice only you can make.

But if rocking your natural hair is important to you, you'll have to make an investment in yourself. Yes, deep conditioning once or twice a week, moisturizing and sealing your hair on a daily basis and styling your natural hair will take time. But so does anything worth having.

I've tried out a number of diets and intense exercise programs, from Weight Watchers to Insanity to P90X. I took the time to write down what I ate every day. I made the time to fit my workouts into my busy schedule. I wanted the results so I did what it took to get them. If you really want to grow healthy, natural hair, then you'll make the time. I promise you won't regret it.

I recommend that you figure out in advance how much time you can devote each week to taking care of your hair and educating yourself about your hair. I also recommend that you schedule your "hair time" by noting it on your calendar or in your natural hair journal. At the start of your journey, the learning process will require more time. But as the learning curve begins to flatten out, you'll be able to reduce that time significantly.

Commitment

In addition to time, you're going to need to be committed to the process. It will take time and experimentation to learn *your* hair and what products respond best to it. There will be times when you are completely frustrated with your hairstyle or disappointed at the slow rate of growth. Transitioning to natural hair is not going to happen overnight. Hair growth takes time. Particularly if your hair is damaged or if you're trying to grow out a relaxer. It will also take a bit of trial and error to find the right products and natural styles that work best for you.

So when you get frustrated and overwhelmed and think about giving up, don't!

Think about the last diet or exercise program you started but didn't finish. Somewhere along the line, you got fed up with the slow results and grabbed the nearest bag of chips or Snickers bar (at least I did). Now think about the last diet or exercise program that you successfully completed. How good did you feel after reaching your goal?

Learning how to care for your natural hair is something you're doing for yourself. You deserve it. So make the commitment and stick with it no matter what.

Patience

This is the most important tool of all! The beautiful, natural hair you want isn't going to happen overnight. It's going to take a lot of patience on your part to get there. Along the way, there will be both successes and failures. Products you love. Products you purchase after watching a tutorial on YouTube that end up being a complete waste of your money. Products that work fabulously for a few months, then suddenly don't work anymore.

But stick with it and somewhere along your journey, you'll find out what works best for you and your hair and the results you desire will begin to materialize. At times, the journey will seem painstakingly slow. If you work through the frustration and stick with it, I guarantee you the rewards will be fabulous. So practice patience! You won't regret it!

Please keep in mind that you won't learn everything you need to know about your natural hair journey overnight. *Kinky Coily: A Natural Hair Resource Guide* is not intended to be a definitive guide on caring for natural hair. It's merely a list of resources to help you begin your own hair care education, which never truly ends. I'm learning new things about my hair every single day.

My ultimate goal in writing this book is to educate, enlighten and empower you to take charge of your own natural hair care. No matter what questions you may have, I'm confident that one or more of the resources identified in this book can provide the answers you're looking for.

Reading this book, however, isn't going to instantly make your natural hair journey fast or easy. We don't all have the same hair types and curl patterns. So what worked for me, may not work for you. You'll have to do your own research to identify the techniques and products that work best for *you* and *your* hair.

Just think of this process as working toward a degree. Reading *Kinky Coily: A Natural Hair Resource Guide* and acting on the information it provides are akin to taking your first college class: Natural Hair Care 101. There's a lot more work to be done before you earn your natural hair care degree. I'm just opening the classroom door.

I wish you much success in discovering the true beauty of your kinky coils.

Good luck and enjoy the journey!

CHAPTER 3

The Journey

WHEN MY FRIEND ALISA FIRST mentioned that she was on a *hair journey*, I had no idea what she was talking about. Now, some three years into my own journey, I consider the word *journey* more than appropriate for this experience.

To take a journey is to travel from one place to another. On my journey, I traveled from a place of unhappiness and despair over the condition of my thinning, damaged hair to a place of wonder and appreciation of my God-given natural hair texture. Where will your journey lead? That's totally up to you. But if you follow the three-step process below, you'll definitely get there.

STEP ONE
Master the Fundamentals of Natural Hair Care

Today, women of color who choose to go natural are learning to care for their hair in ways that differ drastically from the way cosmetologists have been taught to care for our hair. So transitioning to natural hair will mean unlearning what you've been taught about caring for your hair.

Let's begin by discussing some of the most common natural hair care terms and methods you'll need to know. Fasten your seat belts. There's a lot to take in!

The Natural Hair Lingo

Going natural isn't going to just mean a whole new world of hair care, but a whole new language as well. Here are a few of the more common terms you're likely to run across as you begin your natural hair journey. It's not exhaustive, but is sufficient to make you sound like a real naturalista at the next party you attend.

As for the resources I've cited, I've only listed a few articles, books and videos that I have personally read or watched. There are thousands of them on YouTube and the Internet, so don't limit yourself to the ones I've highlighted below. Supplement them with your own research.

ACV

Apple cider vinegar is an excellent product for clarifying your hair. Repeated use of products such as gels and creams can cause buildup on the hair. Rinsing your hair with a solution made up of apple cider vinegar and water will get rid of the buildup.

> *Resource: See my Apple Cider Vinegar Clarifying Rinse recipe on page 132. Also search YouTube for "natural hair" and "ACV" for additional recipes.*

baggying

Baggying helps trap moisture in the hair. The process involves sectioning off the hair and adding a moisturizer to each section, focusing on the ends. The ends are then covered with a small, plastic baggy, held in place by a rubber band. If the hair is too short for sectioning or covering the ends, a plastic shower cap can be used.

> *Resource: Check out "What is the Baggy Method?" by Tia of Her Best Hair at CurlyNikki. com.*

banding

Banding is a way to combat the shrinkage of natural hair after it dries. Kinky hair, when dry, can shrink up to 50% to 70% of its length when wet. You can stretch the hair by banding it, *i.e.*, wrapping it in bands to stretch it out without the use of heat or flat irons.

Resource: Check out blogger BlackOnyx77's YouTube video, "Banding Natural Hair to Stretch No Head, Tutorial Pt.1 and Pt. 2."

big chop

The big chop is the process of cutting off your chemically processed hair (or damaged hair) so that you are *au natural*. Rather than waiting for a relaxer to grow out to start their natural hair journey, many women opt to just cut it off and start over fresh.

Resource: You can find videos on the pros and cons of the big chop on YouTube. Also search CurlyNikki.com and BlackgirlLongHair.com for more discussion on the topic.

breakage vs. shedding

When I started my hair journey, I didn't understand the difference between hair breakage and hair shedding. Shedding is a normal process (provided it's not excessive). We all shed hair on a daily basis. Breakage is not normal and can be caused by such things as heat damage, a lack of moisture, a protein deficiency or even a poor diet. How do you tell the difference between breakage and shedding? When your hair sheds, it sheds from the root, which means you'll see the white bulb on the root. Hair breakage doesn't happen from the root. You'll see broken pieces of hair without the white bulb on the end of the strand.

> **Resource:** *The Science of Black Hair: A Comprehensive Guide to Textured Hair Care by Audrey Davis-Sivasothy, Chapter 6, Protein & Moisture Balancing Strategies for Breakage Correction and Defense.*

clarify

Clarifying your hair is the process of cleansing it to eliminate product buildup, dirt and oils. There are specific shampoos made for clarifying the hair. Using a mixture of water and apple cider vinegar (*see* my Apple Cider Vinegar Clarifying Rinse recipe on page 132) is also a popular clarifying method for many naturals.

> **Resource:** *For an informative article about clarifying, read "When Co-Washing is Not Enough...5 Signs You Need To Do A Clarifying Shampoo" by The Natural Haven on BlackGirlLongHair.com.*

co-wash (low poo or no poo)

Co-washing (also known as low poo or no poo, as in no shampoo) is the process of washing your hair with conditioner. Yes, I know that sounds crazy. It sounded crazy to me too—at first. But what I learned in my early natural hair care research is that most shampoos contain harsh chemicals that are not good for kinky-textured hair. I challenge you to go to your bathroom right now (and also examine the shampoo bottle the next time you visit your hair stylist) and check the label for the chemical *sodium laureth sulfate*. Unless the product is a sulfate-free shampoo, it's probably there. Sodium laureth sulfate is the chemical that makes the shampoo form suds. It is also used in detergents and degreasers. When used on the hair it strips away the natural oils. That is why a conditioner is recommended after shampooing to add back the moisture that the shampoo strips away.

It took me a few weeks to get comfortable with not using shampoo to wash my hair. After co-washing three or four times, I actually went back to my shampoo and that's when I *got it*. My hair felt noticeably rough after rinsing out the shampoo. But after washing it with conditioner, it felt smooth and, yes, clean.

After nearly three years of co-washing, however, I started using a sulfate-free shampoo and only co-wash occasionally. Why? When I was transitioning and wearing my hair underneath a wig, co-washing was great. But when I started shingling my hair and applying gels up to three times a week, I really needed a shampoo (as opposed to a conditioner) to cleanse the product from my hair. You can review my original and current hair regimens on page 114.

> **Resource:** *Check out the following article on co-washing at CurlyNikki.com: "Co-Washing Natural Hair...Is Your Conditioner Good Enough" by TheManeObjective. You'll also find tons of talk about the pros and cons of co-washing on YouTube.*

deep conditioning

Deep conditioning is a special treatment for the hair intended to add moisture and shine, as well as strengthen the hair. Kinky-textured hair tends to be dry and, therefore, needs added moisture. Deep conditioning is especially important for damaged hair as it can make the hair less susceptible to breakage. Using a deep conditioning product with a heat cap will help seal in the moisture.

> *Resource: You can find a boatload of videos on YouTube that discuss deep conditioning products, recipes and processes. Just search for the phrases "natural hair" and "deep conditioning." Of course, CurlyNikki.com and BlackGirlLongHair.com are two additional resources to search.*

defining your curls

Defining your curls is a way to accentuate your natural curls and keep them in place (defined) even after your hair dries. When I wash my hair with conditioner, my hair immediately forms into tight curls. But once it's dry, the curls are gone, replaced by hair that looks cotton-like and curl-less. To define my curls, (*i.e.,* to maintain the curl pattern that emerges when my hair is wet) I have to apply a gel that effectively *defines* my curls. That works for *my* hair texture. Other women with thicker or kinkier hair may need to use a cream or butter and twist their hair to define their curls.

Resource: For instructions on defining your hair, search YouTube for "natural hair" and one of the following terms: "shingling," "twist-out," or "defining curls." You can also check out my video, "How to Shingle Your Hair," on my YouTube Channel, Kinky Coily Pamela.

detangling

Detangling kinky-textured hair after washing can be a big-time hassle, especially for women who have a lot of length. It's important, however, to be gentle and patient during this process to avoid added stress on the hair, which can lead to breakage. Use a wide-toothed comb or your fingers to detangle your hair. Using the right conditioner for your hair (one that tends to be more slippery) can also make the detangling process a breeze.

Resource: Blogger Naputural85 has a great tutorial on detangling natural hair, "How to Detangle Thick, Curly Natural Hair." You'll find it on her YouTube Channel.

diffuser

A diffuser is a flat, circular nozzle with short prongs placed on the end of a blow dryer that allows the hair to be dried without disturbing your curls, which would happen if you dried your hair with just the open nozzle of the hair dryer. The diffuser is used in a plumping motion. When I diffuse my hair, I also hold my head upside down. This adds more volume. Be sure to protect your hair from heat damage by using a blow dryer with a cool setting.

> ***Resource:*** *For a demonstration of diffusing the hair, check out BlackOnyx77's YouTube video "How to Use a Diffuser for Great Curls on Natural Hair." Taren Guy's "Tips on Diffusing" is also another great YouTube video to watch.*

dusting

Dusting is a way to give your ends a light trim, about ¼ inch or less. To dust, twist your hair into several sections (wet or dry), so that you can see the ragged ends, then snip them off. It's called dusting because you're cutting off such a small amount of hair that it looks like dust on the floor. There is disagreement among naturals as to how often the hair should be trimmed. Some argue every three months or so, others say only when needed. How often you trim or dust will depend on the condition of your hair and how you feel about cutting it.

> ***Resource:*** *For instructions on how to dust your ends, check out NaturalMe4C's YouTube video on dusting: "Natural Hair4C-Dusting and Trimming Ends." Also watch "How to Trim Curly Natural Hair" by YouTube blogger Naptural85.*

henna

I am a big fan of henna treatments. Henna is a plant-based powder that is green in color and smells like freshly cut grass. I like the shine it gives my hair, as well as the way it strengthens and covers my gray when I add indigo powder. I also have a very tight curl pattern, which is loosened by henna treatments. Many naturals recommend using body art quality henna.

> **Resource:** *For a thorough explanation of the benefits of henna as well as henna products and a great FAQ on henna, visit Hennaforhair.com. The site also has a video showing how to apply henna. For a henna recipe and application instructions, see Better Than Good Hair: The Curly Girl Guide to Healthy, Gorgeous Natural Hair! by Nikki Walton and Ernessa T. Carter, Chapter Three, The Terrible Twos: Standing By Your Hair Even When It's Acting a Fool.*

line of demarcation

If you have a relaxer, the line of demarcation is the place where your hair's natural texture meets your hair's relaxed texture. Because of the two different hair textures—one kinky, one straight—this area is much more prone to breakage and needs to be handled with tender loving care during the transitioning process.

> **Resource:** *See Hairstylings101's YouTube video "What is Demarcation Line/Point for Hair? (...and Breakage?)."*

LOC method

LOC stands for *liquid, oil, cream.* This is a process for moisturizing and sealing your hair, which I did nightly at the start of my hair journey because my hair was so damaged. The effort definitely paid off. Nowadays, I will use the LOC method once a week, and more often if my hair feels dry.

To do the LOC method, divide your hair into multiple small sections. Apply a liquid, an oil, and a cream to each section, then two-strand twist the section. This process really helped my hair stay moisturized. I currently use either water or a conditioner with a lot of slip (more liquidy as opposed to thick and creamy) as my liquid (Trader Joes Nourish Spa conditioner is one of my favorites). I use grape seed oil or jojoba oil as my oil, and As I Am Double Butter Cream as my cream. You will need to experiment to find out which products work best for your hair. Carrier oils such as olive oil, coconut oil and jojoba oil work best to seal in moisture.

> ***Resource:*** *For instructions on using the LOC method, search "natural hair" and "LOC method" on YouTube. The video "LOC Method-Sealing the Moisture in Your Hair" by BlackOnyx77, is a good one to start with.*

low-manipulation hairstyles

A low-manipulation style is one that avoids excessive handling of the hair in order to avoid breakage. Kinky hair tends to be fragile and very susceptible to breakage, so the more you leave your hair alone when it comes to styling, the better off it will be. Low-manipulation styles don't require the daily use of combs, brushes, curling irons or blow dryers. Wearing your hair in a bun is an example of a low-manipulation hairstyle. Shingling your hair (which is my preferred style) is *not* a low manipulation style because it requires excessive handling of the hair.

> ***Resource:*** *Blogger CharyJay has a ton of videos on YouTube featuring fabulously creative protective styles. Check her out.*

moisture/protein balance

Healthy hair must maintain a proper balance of moisture and protein, otherwise breakage will occur. Moisture deficiency can be caused by things like heat styling and harsh shampoos. Protein deficiency can result from the use of excessive deep conditioning and chemical treatments such as relaxers and hair coloring. Moisture-starved hair is typically brittle and easily broken. Protein-deficient hair is usually limp and stretches easily.

Here's a test for determining whether your hair might need more protein. When your hair is wet, does it feel limp and gummy? If you try to stretch it, does it stretch even more before it finally breaks. This may be an indication that you need more protein.

On the other hand, if your hair when wet doesn't have much stretch and feels rough and brittle and breaks easily, that may be a sign that you need more moisture.

Resource: The Science of Black Hair: A Comprehensive Guide to Textured Hair Care by Audrey Davis-Sivasothy, Chapter 6, Protein & Moisture Balancing Strategies for Breakage Correction and Defense.

moisturizing and sealing

Moisturizing and sealing is the process of using one product to moisturize your hair and a different product (usually an oil) to seal the moisture in. Using the LOC method (*see* page 47) is a process for moisturizing and sealing. It's particularly important to tend to the ends of the hair, which is the oldest part of the hair and needs the most tender loving care, especially for those who want to retain length.

Resource: For tips on moisturizing and sealing, you'll find more articles and videos than you'll ever need on YouTube, CurlyNikki.com and BlackGirlLongHair.com

oils (essential and carrier)

There are two types of oils that are great for your hair: essential oils (*e.g.,* rosemary, peppermint and tea tree oils) and carrier oils (*e.g.,* jojoba, coconut and olive oils). Essential oils contain the *essence* of the plant from which the oils are derived and are great for stimulating hair growth and treating scalp conditions. Carrier oils *carry* the essential oils onto the scalp.

Resource: For a great article about essential and carrier oils, including a summary of the specific benefits of the various oils, read "Oils Explained: Essential Oils and Carrier Oils For Hair" at BlackHair101.com.

pH balance

The potential of hydrogen, or pH, is the measurement of how acidic or alkaline a substance is. Healthy hair has a pH balance between 4.5 and 5.5. This natural hair acidity prevents the growth of fungi and bacteria in the hair and scalp, and keeps the cuticle closed and healthy. It's important to use products that don't disrupt the natural pH of your hair. A product that is too alkaline will cause the hair cuticle to open, while a substance that is too acidic will cause the cuticle to contract.

Resource: For information on how to determine the pH balance of your hair products, see The Science of Black Hair: A Comprehensive Guide to Textured Hair Care, by Audrey Davis-Sivasothy Chapter 2, Textured Hair Properties & Principles. Also check out Kimmaytube's informative four-part YouTube series on hair structure, starting with "Structure of the Hair – Part 1 – The Basics."

pineappling

Pineappling is a way to protect your hair during sleep to preserve your curls. Gather your curls high on top of your head into a loose ponytail and tie it with a Scrunchie (thus, resembling a pineapple). Wrap your hair around the sides with a silk or satin scarf, leaving the hair loose on top of your head. This process works best for those with length and helps to keep your second-day curls (or third or fourth-day curls) vibrant and frizz-free.

> **Resource:** *See the article "Back to Pineappling-My Nighttime Regimen" by Curly Nikki at CurlyNikki.com.*

porosity

Porosity refers to how porous your hair is. In other words, how well it absorbs moisture. Understanding whether you have low or high-porosity hair (or somewhere in the middle) is important for selecting the right products for your hair.

> **Resources:** *For an excellent summary on porosity, including how to determine if you have low or high-porosity hair, consult The Science of Black Hair: A Comprehensive Guide to Textured Hair Care by Audrey Davis-Sivasothy, Chapter 2, Textured Hair Properties & Principles. Also check out the YouTube video "Question of the Day/FAQ: Porosity and Natural Hair" by blogger Quest for the Perfect Curl (Elle) for another great discussion about porosity.*

pre-poo

Pre-poo means to condition your hair *before* you wash it. My hair mentor Deanie was the first person I ever heard use this term. Part of her recipe for helping me repair my damaged hair included applying a deep conditioner and oils on my dry, unwashed hair, preferably with a heat cap for better penetration. Pre-pooing is intended to prepare the hair for the shampooing process, which can strip the hair of moisture as well as its natural oils. Pre-pooing helps maintain the moisture kinky hair so desperately needs.

> ***Resource:*** *For some great pre-poo recipes, search YouTube for "natural hair" and "pre-poo."*

product junkie

A product junkie is someone who loves to roam the aisles of beauty supply stores and cannot resist trying a new product. I've been struggling with this addiction for some time. If you loiter in the aisles of beauty supply stores and walk out with five or more products per visit when you went in for one, you might be a product junkie.

> ***Resource:*** *If you don't believe that I'm a product junkie, check out the photograph of my product stash!*

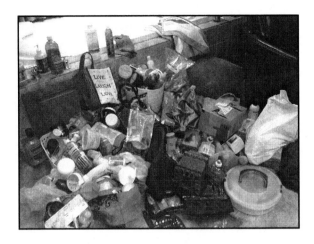

protective hairstyles

A protective style is one that protects your edges, the nape of your neck and the end of your hair (the oldest part of the hair). During my transitioning period, I wore a wig as my protective style. My goal was to reduce exposure and stress on my hair to prevent further breakage. Other protective styles include wearing your hair in a bun (provided you have enough length) or cornrows.

> ***Resource:*** *For some great protective styles check out bloggers CharyJay and MsVaughnTV on YouTube.*

refreshing

Refreshing refers to the process of reviving a natural hairstyle so that it looks almost as fresh as the day it was first done. This usually requires adding water or a moisturizer to add some life to your curls. Organic Root Stimulator's Curls Unleashed Second Chance Curl Refresher is a great product for reviving second-day hair.

> **Resource:** *See the video "Nighttime Routine and Refreshing My Wash and Go for Natural Hair" by YouTube Blogger Quest for the Perfect Curl (Elle).*

retaining length

Retaining length refers to the process of preventing hair from breaking so that it can continue to grow. Two keys to retaining length are proper moisture and protecting the ends of the hair. Many kinky-textured women don't believe that they can grow hair past shoulder length. Our natural sisters with hair down their backs have proven that this is a myth.

> **Resource:** *If you really want to see some sisters with length, visit Urbanbushbabes' YouTube channel and soak up their knowledge because they have loads to impart.*

second-day hair

Second (and third and fourth, etc.) day hair refers to how long a style (such as a twist-out) can be maintained before it becomes frizzy and unruly and has to be redone.

> *Resource:* See *"Quick Fishtail Braid Out: Second Day Natural Hair" by YouTube Blogger Naptural85 and "Curlformers on Natural Hair: Second Day Hair with Separated Curls" by YouTube Blogger Mahogany Curls.*

shingling

Shingling is the process of defining curls by using a gel or cream and individually twirling a small section of hair around the finger. This is my staple method of doing my hair and is a form of a wash 'n go. My picture on the cover of this book shows my hair shingled.

> *Resource: See my YouTube channel, Kinky Coily Pamela, and the video "How to Get the Kinky Coily Look" for a demonstration of how I shingle my hair.*

shrinkage

The dreaded shrinkage is the way wet kinky-textured hair draws up after it has dried. Depending on the curl pattern, dry kinky-textured hair can shrink as much as 50% to 70% from its length when wet. I'm a witness!.

> *Resource: For tips on combatting shrinkage, search for "natural hair" and "shrinkage" at BlackGirlLongHair.com, CurlyNikki.com and YouTube.*

sulfates

Sulfates are compounds used in detergents and cleansers that generate suds. The majority of shampoos on the market contain these harsh detergents, which are extremely drying to kinky-textured hair. Most shampoos contain a sulfate such as sodium laureth sulfate, sodium lauryl sulfate or ammonium lauryl sulfate. One of the reasons conditioners are recommended after shampooing is because shampoos strip the hair of its natural oils and conditioners are needed to restore moisture. Start reading labels. If you see the word *sulfate*, you may want to pass on the product. Luckily, more sulfate-free shampoos are hitting the market.

> **Resource:** *See The Science of Black Hair: A Comprehensive Guide to Textured Hair Care by Audrey Davis-Sivasothy, Chapter 5, Healthy Hair Management.*

TWA

Once I began my journey, I searched high and low for a definition of TWA, which naturals on YouTube tossed around with regularity. About a month later, I came across an article that defined the acronym. A TWA is a teeny weeny afro. This is what's left after the big chop!

> **Resource:** *Search YouTube for "natural hair" and "TWA." It's fun to check out the progress photos of women who did the big chop. The subsequent hair growth of Mahogany Curls and*

Naptural85 after their big chops was stunning. Check them out on YouTube.

twist out

A twist out is a natural hair styling technique that involves twisting the hair (either wet or dry) in separate sections then untwisting them after they are dry for a full natural style. The two-strand twist is one of the most popular twist outs. For the best styles, many women leave their hair twisted for a day or more, then unfurl the twists to reveal a full-textured look.

> *Resource: Check out the YouTube video for "natural hair" and "TWA" by SimplYounique. Her Journey videos are fabulous, as well as motivating!*

wash 'n go

A wash 'n go is using conditioner or a styling product on wet hair to define curls without having to do further styling. I shingle my hair (individually twirl my curls into formation), which is a form of a wash 'n go. Some naturals can simply define their curls using a conditioner. For them, it really is a wash 'n go.

> *Resource: Mahogany Curls has multiple wash 'n go tutorials on YouTube. Start with "Wash 'n Go: Short Natural Hair" and follow her hair growth through "Wash 'n Go: Updated Routine."*

You'll also find tons of videos by simply searching YouTube for "natural hair" and "wash and go."

For additional natural hair care terms, visit Urbanbushbabes.com and click on *Natural Dictionary* under the *Hair* tab. Also check out the *Hair Terminology* page at Hairlista.com.

Tools of the Trade

Going natural requires caring for your hair very differently than you did when you were wearing a pressed or relaxed hairstyle. For one, natural hair is fragile and needs to be handled more delicately. Here are some of the tools you might want to have in your natural hair care arsenal.

afro pic

This is what I use to style my hair after shingling. Once my curls dry, I use the afro pic to lift it for more volume.

blow dryer with diffuser

Heat is generally bad for natural hair, but there will be times when you need to blow dry your hair. Just make sure you select a blow dryer with a cool setting. Many blow dryers now come with a diffuser, which allows you to plump your hair to add volume.

comb (wide-toothed)

As you go natural, you'll learn that carefully detangling your hair is one way to avoid breakage. When detangling your hair, a wide tooth comb will be something you can't live without. Or, like some naturals, you may want to detangle with your fingers.

Denman brush
This little brush can help detangle and also be used to shingle the hair. It looks like a typical brush but has plastic teeth.

hair clips
You will need to section your hair when doing certain hairstyles. Hair clips will make this process easier.

hair steamer
This is more of a treat than a necessity. I didn't purchase a steamer until more than a year into my hair journey. It's been the one thing that helps my hair retain moisture. I love my steamer and wish I'd purchased it earlier. Check out my video, *The Joy of Steaming Your Natural Hair* on my YouTube Channel Kinky Coily Pamela.

heat cap
A heat cap will help seal in the moisture in your hair when you're deep conditioning.

hooded dryer
To deep condition or to speed up the drying time of your twist out, a hooded dryer is good to have. Just make sure it also has a cool setting and/or a low heat setting.

lint-free towel (or old T-shirt)

As a natural, you'll need to be gentle with your hair. Rather than using a linen towel to dry my just-washed hair, I use a soft, microfiber (lint-free) towel, which is less likely to cause friction that can create breakage. An old white, extra-large T-shirt also works well. Cut off the sleeves, then cut it down the middle.

plastic bonnets (disposable)

You'll need plastic bonnets when you condition your hair. Save your money up front and get more bang for your buck by purchasing the 100 pack. You'll need them.

containers

spray bottle

Some of the products you mix up will work better if you spray them onto your hair. You'll also need a bottle to spray water on your hair for moisture.

tint bottle

I recommend purchasing the plastic bottles with the pointy tips used for tinting hair. Purchase the ones with the measurement markings on the side. Buy three or four. As you begin to mix various oils and products, you'll need them.

large containers with tops

You may want to create some of your own products and you'll need a container to store them. Rather than buy them, I use the empty margarine tubs and also keep the squeeze bottles after I run out of a product.

plastic or latex gloves
If you color or use henna on your hair, you'll definitely need gloves to protect your hands and nails from staining.

satin/silk scarf, bonnet or pillowcase
Protecting your hair while you sleep at night is as important as protecting it during the day. To avoid friction that can cause breakage, never wrap your natural hair with cotton fabric. A satin or silk bonnet, scarf or pillowcase will protect your natural hair.

Now that you know the natural hair lingo and the tools you'll need, let's discuss hair textures and curl patterns.

Understanding Hair Texture and Curl Patterns

As you begin to care for your own hair, you will become intimately familiar with it. By this, I mean that you will become accustomed to how it feels. You will know instantly if your hair likes a product or hates it. You will learn whether creams or gels are best for defining your curls. Before you get to this point, however, it's important to understand your hair type.

Kinky hair, though it appears coarse, is actually fragile and breaks easily. It can also be dry which further makes it prone to breakage. We don't all have the same hair type, which means a product that works for me, may not work for you. It will take time and experimentation to find out what works best for you.

It's a good idea to know both your hair texture and curl pattern. Your curl pattern is how your kinky curls form. Your hair texture is the thickness of your individual strands: fine, medium or thick. I've heard the following definitions for hair texture. If your hair is thinner than a piece of thread, it's fine. If it's about the same width as a thread, it's medium. If it's thicker than a piece of thread, it's thick. My hair is fine, though it looks thick because of the style I wear.

One of the most often-quoted guides for identifying hair types was created by celebrity stylist Andre Walker, Oprah's long-time hair stylist. His system categorizes hair types from 1a to 4c (*i.e.*, 1a, 1b, 1c, 2a, 2b, 2c, etc.) Here's a more simplified summary of his system: Type 1 is straight hair (no curl or wave pattern); Type 2 is wavy hair (long S-shaped curls); Type 3 is curly hair (more defined S-shaped curls); and Type 4 is kinky hair (tight coils with more of a Z- or corkscrew-shaped pattern). Visit the resources below and take a look at photographs of the various hair types, then take a look at your own hair to decide where you fall.

There is much debate over whether we can or even should categorize our hair types. But don't stress over it. While I'm pretty certain that I'm a 4, I don't know for sure whether I'm a 4a, 4b or 4c. I do know, however, that my hair is kinky and is very tightly coiled. Shingling my hair works well for me precisely because I have a tight, springy curl pattern.

> ***Resources:*** *The website BlackGirlLongHair.com features a great article on hair types, complete with photographs of women who fit each category. To find the article, type "Natural Hair Type Guide: Which Type Are You?" in the website's search box. The website NaturallyCurly.com also has an informative article on curl patterns. Click on the "Hair Types" tab on the Home page, then under "Texture Typing," click on "Curl Pattern." This site also shows pictures of the various curl patterns.*
>
> *You can find an informative summary on hair types in The Science of Black Hair: A Comprehensive Guide to Textured Hair Care by Audrey Davis-Sivasothy, Chapter 2, Textured Hair Properties & Principles. Finally, Curly Girl: The Handbook by Lorraine Massey also has an excellent discussion on hair types and curl patterns in Chapter 3, Identifying Your Curl Type. Also read Chapter 6, Multi-Cultural Hair. And you can always conduct a search on YouTube for "natural hair" and "hair types" or "curl patterns" for more helpful information.*

Identifying Your Curl Pattern

Once you're armed with an understanding of the different curl types, here's a technique that will help you identify your own.

First, wash your hair. While it's wet, take a section in the front and apply a creamy conditioner (VO5, Suave or Herbal Essence will work). Does a wave or curl pattern emerge? Separate out a few strands so you can clearly see how or if your hair curls. Take a picture so you can refer to it later and compare it to the curl patterns on the resources listed above. Depending on your hair texture, once your hair dries, you may find that your curl pattern is not as defined as it was when your hair was wet. In order to maintain a curly style after your hair dries, you'll need to define your curls by using a gel or cream or a twisting method (such as a two-strand twist). For experimental purposes only, apply a heavy gel like Eco Styler Gel to a small section of your hair. When I use the Eco Styler Gel on my semi-wet hair, a curl pattern does emerge and once it's dry, although my curls have shrunk, my curl pattern is well-defined. Check out my video *How to Determine Your Curl Pattern* by visiting my YouTube Channel, Kinky Coily Pamela.

After trying multiple times to get a decent twist-out, I finally faced the reality that a twist out probably won't look good on my hair until I have more length. My hair isn't very thick, so once I've unfurled the twists, I look like I stuck my finger in an electrical socket. But when I shingle my hair using a gel, I get the full curly look that is pictured on the cover of this book.

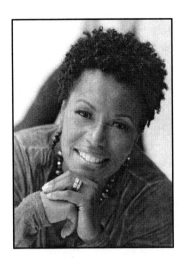

By contrast, my friend Karen Copeland has thick coarse hair. When she tried the same gel I use, it did not define her curl pattern. In order to get her fantastic look, she needs a cream rather than a gel and does a two-strand twist.

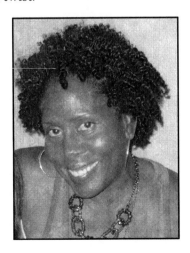

Again, I think that knowing your hair type and curl pattern is a good thing. But stressing out because you can't precisely pinpoint your hair type (3a, 4c, etc.) is *not* a good thing.

One more point. You should be aware that your curl pattern may not be the same all over your head. My curl pattern is extremely tight in the back, loose at the crown and medium-tight everywhere else.

Selecting The Right Hair Care Products

The success of your natural hair journey will depend a great deal on finding the right products. Without the right products, you won't get the look you want and, therefore, you're more likely to abandon your journey. I have friends who have tried to go natural and I mean *tried* with a little *t*. They apply one or two products to their hair, then give up, complaining that "I just can't wear my hair natural!"

If you really want to rock your natural hair, you'll have to do the work to find the right products for your hair. I can suggest a thousand things, but you'll have to do the research and experimentation to find out what works best for you and your hair. Yes, it's frustrating to buy a product that works on your friend but leaves you looking like a greasy mess. Been there, done that. But when you find that product that works like a charm, it's hallelujah time!

Learn to be a Label Reader

The discussion above about hair texture and curl patterns will play a role in the hair care products you select for your hair. In the beginning, I bought anything and everything and wasted a lot of money in the process. Late one night I watched six YouTube videos raving about a new curl-enhancing gel. Always on the lookout for something new and better, I ripped off my pajamas, jumped into my jeans and drove to three different drug stores before I found it. Did it work for me? Nope. Thank goodness it was only a few bucks.

So my advice is to be discerning with the products you buy. (Do as I say, not as I do.) Also, you must decide whether you intend to go *all the way* natural. I know naturals who only put truly natural products on their hair. Simply because something says "natural" on the label, however, doesn't mean that it is. Most of the products these women use are whipped up in their kitchens because they don't want chemicals *of any kind* to touch their tresses. If being a *bona fide* natural means only using all-natural products, then I don't meet the test. There are chemicals I try to avoid, but I don't have the time or the desire to mix up everything that goes on my hair. You will have to make that decision. If you do want to be a true natural, you'll find the following books helpful:

- *The Kitchen Beautician: Natural Hair Care Recipes for Beautiful Healthy Hair* by Dezarae Henderson.

- *Coif Cuisine: Natural Hair Recipes & Side Dishes for the Natural Hair and Now* by Candace O. Kelley.

- *55 Fun & Fabulous DIY Beauty Recipes: Natural Homemade Skin, Hair, & Nail Care Recipes Using Aromatherapy Essential Oils (Holistic Tips, Recipes & Remedies Series)* by Amy Waldow.

- *Natural Hair Care for Curls and Kinks* by Todra Payne.

Also check out the fantastic natural recipes posted by YouTube blogger Naptural85.

Okay, just because I buy products rather than make them doesn't mean I'll put any old thing in my hair. There are some products, chemicals and ingredients that we need to be wary of. I've listed below a few ingredients that many naturals consider a no-no. I *try* to avoid them, but if my hair seems to love a particular product that might have one of these ingredients, I go with what works for *my* hair. (You'll know if your hair loves a product by the way it behaves when you use it.) I've also listed some ingredients you definitely *want* to see in your hair care products.

Ingredients to Avoid

- **Sulfates**
  Sulfates are a category of foaming agents (also known as surfactants) found in shampoos. These harsh detergents rob your hair of the moisture that

kinky-texture hair desperately needs. Look for ingredients with the word *sulfate* in it, such as sodium lauryl *sulfate*, sodium laureth *sulfate*, and ammonium lauryl *sulfate*, and avoid these products.

- **Alcohol**
  Alcohol is particularly drying for kinky-textured hair. Make every effort to avoid products with alcohol.

- **Petroleum**
  Petroleum sits on the hair, repelling other products, preventing the hair from getting the moisture it needs. Would you put motor oil in your hair? Enough said.

- **Mineral Oil**
  Mineral oil is a petroleum-based oil which coats the hair, preventing other products you use from penetrating the hair shaft. It also clogs the pores of the scalp, which interfere with the creation of your natural oils, thus leading to breakage.

Ingredients to Look For

- **Water**
  Water is a natural moisturizer. Kinky-textured hair is prone to dryness. Water will help restore moisture. When reading product labels, when the first ingredient listed is water, that's a good start.

- **Aloe Vera**
  Aloe vera, a plant-based gel, helps to restore the scalp's pH balance. It also hydrates and conditions the hair and scalp, which aids in hair growth.

- **Vegetable Glycerin**
  Glycerin adds a layer of oil over the hair, which helps to lock in moisture.

- **Shea Butter**
  Hair butters, like shea butter, help to restore moisture to the hair. Butters in general are good for kinky-textured hair because they help to seal in the moisture.

Consult Product Reviews and Tutorials

You should also consult the ton of product reviews and tutorials on the Internet and YouTube. When naturals find products they like, they love to tell the world about it. So scour YouTube for the product you're thinking about trying out or the category of products you want more information about. You should also visit online forums for recommendations. I highly recommend browsing any customer reviews for the product, if available.

Talk to Friends and Strangers

If you have friends and family members who are natural, you're probably already sharing product knowledge. If not, get with it. And don't be afraid to approach a stranger. Us naturals are some of the friendliest people on the planet and we *love* to talk about hair. I learned about the No. 1 can't-live-without product in my hair care arsenal (Uncle Funky's Daughter Curly Magic) from a stranger I met at a dinner party. Of course, two naturals sitting next to each other can't help but talk about hair. Strangers often come up to me to ask about the products I use. So keep an eye out for other naturals and use them as resources.

Keep an Accurate Record of the Products You Use

It's a good idea to make a note of products that work or don't work for you in your journal. I've tried so many things that sometimes I forget what I purchased. So now I refer to my journal before trying something new because there's a good chance I've already tried it. I can't count how many times I came home with a product that I'd tried months ago and hated.

Exercise Caution When Trying Out a New Product

By exercising caution, I mean make sure the new product you tried really works the way you think it does before committing to it. Avoid trying a new product in the morning before heading off to work. I'm always trying out new curl-defining gels. A few months ago, I found one that gave me super-defined curls. I first tried it on a Monday morning and left the house looking good and feeling great. A couple of hours later, when my hair had completely dried, I was ready to scratch my scalp off! The gel had dried hard, making my scalp itch and leaving white flakes all over my head. I rushed off to the ladies room to try to get rid of the flaking, but that only made it worse. It was very embarrassing to have a co-worker come up to me and ask, "What's that white stuff in your hair?" I had to head home during the lunch hour to wash it out. So test out those new products over the weekend when you don't have any place to go.

Pay Attention to Your Hair's Likes and Dislikes

Pay attention to the products your hair likes and doesn't like. During my strict co-washing days, I was always trying out new conditioners, but time after time, I always went back to my old standby, Herbal Essence's Hello Hydration. For whatever reason, my hair loves being co-washed with that conditioner. I can feel my hair soften in ways that it doesn't with other conditioners, and definitely not with shampoo. I've also heard other naturals rave about how much their hair loves coconut oil. I've tried it—repeatedly—but I don't like the way my hair feels during and after a coconut oil application. But it's a much different story with jojoba oil and grape seed oil. I can immediately feel the difference. So listen to your hair. It's talking to you.

Experiment but Don't Become a Product Junkie

Being willing to experiment with products and hair styles is one of the most important things you can do to ensure that your hair journey is a successful one. You'll learn a lot from the books you read and the bloggers you follow. And if you're anything like me, you'll be excited about all the possibilities for your hair. Enjoy the journey. But place a limit on your experimentation or you'll end up wasting a lot of money.

You can see from the photograph of my personal natural hair arsenal on page 53 that I've experimented with lots of products. I admit it. I'm a product junkie. I now love shopping for hair products more than I enjoy shopping for clothes or shoes. (Really, I do!) I'm so excited when I run across a new product line to try out. Sometimes it works out great, sometimes it doesn't. I can remember stepping into my local Sally's Beauty Supply and right there on the shelf facing me as I walked in was a new product line I had never seen before: As I Am. I immediately bought four of the products. As it turned out I liked all of them, but I *loved* As I Am's Double Butter Cream. To this day, it is my favorite cream for moisturizing my hair. I've tried others, but I always go back to my Double Butter.

The same thing happened when I stumbled upon Taliah Waajid's Black Earth natural hair products in my local CVS. I was so excited to find yet another natural hair care company, so I had to try them out. I wasn't disappointed. The African Healing Oyl is now one of my staples.

But there are dangers associated with being a product junkie. You can't use *everything*. Trying too many different products on your hair can be confusing for you as well as your tresses. How will you know what really works if you use one product one week and a different one two weeks later? It takes time to determine a product's effect on your hair. How long you should give a product will depend on your patience level. I'll admit that I'm often quick to give up on something. But on a few occasions I've returned to a *failed* product only because I was running low on one of my favorites. And surprisingly, in those few instances, what didn't work well before worked out great months later. This may have been due to the fact that the texture and condition of my hair changed as it became healthier. So keep that in mind before you toss a product you don't like.

Thank God for natural hair Meetup groups and product exchanges, where naturals can happily swap or give away products that didn't work out.

Keep Your Journal Up To Date
I began to keep a hair journal very early in my journey. Since I was super-serious about my natural hair journey, I started using the same tracking process I used with my weight loss and exercise programs. Just as I took *before* pictures when I started P9ox, I also took pictures of my damaged hair at the start of my journey. On the one hand, my *before* photographs were quite depressing. On the other hand, they served as a source of motivation. Just as I had faith that Weightwatchers and P9ox would help me eliminate my unwanted pounds, I also had faith that if I did the work, my transition to natural hair would transform my damaged hair into beautiful, healthy hair. And my prayers were indeed answered.

I was also determined to track my progress because I knew that once I had achieved my hair goals, I would have a story to tell. I knew that my *before* and *after* pictures would turn the doubters into believers. (Visit my YouTube Channel, Kinky Coily Pamela, and check out my video, *My Transition to Natural Hair: The First 9 Months* and you'll see what I mean).

For my first journal, I purchased a simple calendar arranged in a monthly format, showing the entire month on two facing pages. I made sure there was enough space to make short notations about what I did to my hair on a given day. I prefer the monthly format because I like to see the entire month at a glance, rather than having to turn the page to see what I did the previous weeks. You can purchase the journal that accompanies this book, *The Kinky Coily Natural Hair Journal* (available at Amazon.com), or create your own.

In my journal I kept an accurate record of when I co-washed, deep-conditioned, colored my gray and trimmed (yes, I trimmed my own hair!). I wrote down the products I used and made notes about what worked and what didn't. My hair journal was effectively a workout program for my hair.

Since there's not a lot of space to write, I used the following abbreviations in my journal:

- W – wash
- CW – co-wash
- DC – deep conditioning
- LOC – liquid, oil, cream
- MS – moisturizing and seal

- PT – protein treatment
- T – trim
- HT – henna treatment
- CG – cover gray

It's a good idea to review your journal each month and analyze whether your regimen is working for you. If not, make some changes. Your journal will also be useful if you run into problems. When I began to experience hair breakage, I took a look back at my hair journal. I could see that over a three-week period I was co-washing my hair every couple of days because I wanted it to look fresh for events I was attending. Well, I immediately suspected that over washing might be the source of my problems. When I cut back on my frequent co-washing, the hair breakage stopped. On another occasion, after finding my hair limp and lifeless, I turned to one of my Go To resources, *The Science of Black Hair: A Comprehensive Guide to Textured Hair Care* by Audrey Davis-Sivasothy, and determined that over-conditioning was the problem. Having my journal to review exactly how I was caring for my hair was crucial in helping me identify my temporary hair woes and correct them.

You don't have to journal forever. In the beginning, I was very diligent about recording my regimen. After about two years natural, I cut back a lot, primarily because I had more confidence about the care of my hair. Decide what works best for you.

Make Water Your BFF

Unlike when you wore your hair straight, water should now be your best friend. Kinky hair needs hydration and water is one of the best sources of it. If you have dry or damaged hair, misting with water and sealing with an oil and/or cream can do wonders to add moisture. When you look for products such as moisturizes and conditioners, water should be listed as one of the first, if not *the* first, ingredient on the list.

A Word About Hair Growth

On average, hair grows at the rate of about ¼ to ½ inch per month. Some people experience more growth, others less. There's a perception that kinky hair cannot grow long, *i.e.*, well past the shoulders. This is a myth. Our hair doesn't grow long because we've been engaged in a vicious cycle of hair growth and breakage. Harsh shampoos, chemicals and excessive heat have contributed to stunting our hair growth. When those elements are removed, and our hair is treated properly (sufficient moisture, avoidance of heat, protective styling) it flourishes and we can attain incredible length. For advice on growing and retaining hair length, check out Urbanbushbabes.com. They are my personal long-hair experts. Also check out *The Science of Black Hair: A Comprehensive Guide to Textured Hair Care* by Audrey Davis-Sivasothy. If you're serious about your hair, I recommend that you read the book from cover to cover. You will learn everything you need to know about kinky-textured hair.

Coloring Natural Hair

I love color, but other than covering my gray, I haven't been daring enough to take that on myself. I recognize that color can be drying to hair and so I'm reluctant to go all out and rock my Rihanna red. I guess I've also had too many disastrous results—both coloring it myself and having it done by a licensed stylist. If I decide to add a little color to my life, I will place my hair in the hands of a natural hair stylist. If you want to go for it, do check out a reputable blogger on YouTube for help. I'd suggest that you begin with Coloured Beautiful. That sister has no problem changing her colors! And of course, do consult the natural hair care Bible, *The Science of Black Hair: A Comprehensive Guide to Textured Hair Care* by Audrey Davis-Sivasothy Chapter 9, Coloring Textured Hair.

To cover my gray, I use henna with indigo powder which gives me an intense black color. When I'm too tired for all the work that goes into mixing the henna, I use Deity America Color Change Shampoo, which according to the label, is a natural, plant based product. I always make sure I deep condition after covering my gray. For more tips on covering gray, search YouTube for *natural hair* and *covering gray*.

Flat Ironing Natural Hair: Beware of Excessive Heat

Many of the bloggers I follow go back and forth between wearing their hair natural and flat-ironed. So, of course, when I decided to wear my hair straightened for New Year's Eve, it never crossed my mind that once I was ready to go back to my kinky coily look, that there might be a problem. Two days later, when I co-washed my hair, four separate sections remained straight at the ends. And I mean bone straight! No amount of washing brought back my curl pattern. If I didn't know better, I would have thought that someone had relaxed my ends while I was asleep. I scoured YouTube and the Internet for answers. Some bloggers recommended washing my hair in non-alcoholic beer. Others said be patient. My curls would resurface in their own time. Most troubling was that some naturals said their curl pattern never came back!

I temporarily used perm rods to curl those straight sections, hoping that my straight ends would ultimately revert to their naturally kinky texture. That didn't happen. Six weeks later, tired of wearing the perm rods, I went to a stylist and had those straight ends clipped off, forcing me to also cut the rest of my hair to make it even.

Why did this happen? In straightening my hair, a very, very hot flat iron was used in order to make it bone straight. Also, no heat protectant was applied to my hair before straightening it. And though I only wore my hair straight for a couple of days, I "touched up" those same sections with my own flat iron a few times, further breaking down my natural curl pattern. I ignored everything I knew about the horrors of excessive heat. Since I only intended to wear my hair straight for a short period of time, I wasn't particularly concerned about the heat. As a result, I paid big for my mistake by having to cut my hair.

I've heard other horror stories of women who were natural for years and found that their hair simply broke off when they flat-ironed it. This discussion is not meant to say that you shouldn't flat iron natural hair. It's meant to say that you *should be careful when flat ironing natural hair and avoid excessive heat.* If I decide to temporarily wear my hair straight again (and at some point I may), I'll make sure it's done by a natural hair stylist who understands the danger of excessive heat.

The Hair Vitamins Debate

For decades, there's been a debate in the medical community about the value of supplements. I take several supplements, including a hair vitamin. Biotin is the main ingredient in vitamins for the hair, skin and nails. Biotin is a water-soluble B vitamin which combats dryness and promotes healthy hair growth by increasing the elasticity of the hair's cortex. It's also believed to help in the transfer of carbon dioxide, which promotes the metabolism of carbohydrates and fat. Biotin is found in egg yolks, meat, fish, dairy products, nuts, and beans. Many naturals consider biotin a staple in their product regimen, including me.

Do You Still Need a Hair Stylist?

Yes! Although you may not make frequent visits, I think it's good to have a professional you can turn to when you have questions or issues with your hair (and you will have them). However, it's essential that you select a stylist who is knowledgeable about natural hair. Many stylists are seeing their customers go natural and are jumping on the bandwagon but some haven't yet acquired sufficient knowledge about caring for natural hair. I met a woman at a party who told me that she was a natural hair stylist. She went on to explain that she does twist-outs and other natural hair styles. I asked her if she uses sulfates and her eyes glazed over. She had no idea what I was talking about. A natural hair stylist is not someone who can do a twist out. It's someone who's knowledgeable about caring for kinky-textured hair.

For anyone in the L.A. area, here are my personal hair care professionals:

Tallulah "Lulu" Marcelin
I Love Lulu Hair Spa
733 S. La Brea Ave
Los Angeles, CA 90036
www.iloveluluhairspa.com
iloveluluhairspa@yahoo.com
(323) 934-5727

I Love Lulu Hair Spa is exactly what the name says, a spa for your hair! Lulu is extremely knowledgeable about natural hair and her salon offers unique treatments that you won't find anyplace else. I love the scalp massage and the Vitamin B5 and steam treatments. And don't forget to check out her handmade products for the hair and body.

Tammy Griffin
Suburban Urban Hair Designs
2292 N. Lincoln Avenue
Altadena, CA 91001
Subhair2@yahoo.com
(626) 676-2723

Tammy is famous for her twists and short haircuts.
You won't find anybody more talented with a pair of
scissors. She did my big chop and I highly recommend her, especially if you've had a bad experience
with a scissor-happy stylist. She's not one of them.
I am thrilled that she is embracing the natural hair
movement.

Shanta Ellis
Emerald Chateau Beauty Salon
401 E Hillcrest Blvd,
Inglewood, CA 90301
braidsbyshanta@yahoo.com
(310) 904-7644

I would call Shanta the baddest braider on the
planet, but I don't want her to get a big head. My
hair grew like crazy in her able hands. If you're
looking for a protective style to help you through
the transitioning process, Shanta will hook you up.

When to Consult a Doctor

There are some hair problems that no amount of self-care will fix. If you're experiencing excessive hair loss or believe your health or diet is impacting the condition of your hair, it's best to consult a medical doctor who specializes in hair loss. It's possible that you could have a condition call alopecia areata, in which the immune system mistakenly attacks the hair follicles. If that's the case, a licensed doctor should be treating you, not a YouTube blogger!

Children and Natural Hair

It's my hope that all the mothers and grandmothers out there are raising their daughters to appreciate their kinky hair and that we no longer have to hear talk about "good hair." The reality is that the versatility of our hair, in my opinion, puts it at the top of the hair chain.

For information on caring for children's natural hair, please consult *The Science of Black Hair: A Comprehensive Guide to Textured Hair Care* by Audrey Davis-Sivasothy. Chapter 12, Regimen-Building Considerations for Kids, discusses the natural hair care needs of children. It contains specific regimen-building considerations for kids from birth to two years as well as toddlers and beyond.

Better Than Good Hair: The Curly Girl Guide to Healthy, Gorgeous Natural Hair! by Nikki Walton and Ernessa T. Carter is another great resource for caring for children's hair. Check out Chapter Five, Natural From The Start: Curly Kids.

You should also search *children* and *natural hair* on YouTube and you'll find loads of helpful videos.

The following children's books use fictional characters to help young girls appreciate their natural hair. They are great for building self-esteem and would all make great gifts for the young natural in your life.

I Love My Natural Hair by Tiffany Anderson (2013). Written by a mother of three who is a natural hair care professional, this children's book follows the journey of a young girl learning to embrace her natural hair. The author wrote the book to encourage girls to be proud of themselves no matter what texture they have.

Color My Fro: A Natural Hair Coloring Book for Big Hair Lovers of All Ages by Crystal Swain-Bates and Janine Carrington.
This entertaining book celebrates the beauty of black women and natural hair. You'll find dozens of natural hair inspired illustrations.

Big Hair, Don't Care by Crystal Swain-Bates and Megan Bair (Illustrator).
In this book, Lola has really big hair, much bigger than the other kids at her school, but that doesn't stop her from telling anyone who will listen just how much she *loves* her hair. Designed to boost self-esteem and build confidence in kids of all races, this beautifully illustrated picture book is aimed at boys and girls who may need a reminder that it's okay to be different.

I Love My Hair! by Natasha Anastasia Tarpley (Author) and E. B. Lewis (Illustrator).
A Blackboard Children's Book of the Year, this whimsical story encourages African-American children to feel good about their special hair and to be proud of their heritage.

My Hair is So Happy by Nik Scott.
Promise, Hope, Grace and Faith all have different hair types, but upon closer inspection they all have one thing in common: curly hair.

STEP TWO
Create Your Natural Hair Care Go To Team

Now that you understand some of the basic requirements of caring for natural hair, you'll need to create your resource team—people and places you can consult for advice and motivation as you commence your natural hair journey. In other words, your Go To Team.

Thanks to technology, you have a wealth of information at your very fingertips. Kinky-textured women all around the globe are freely sharing information about natural hair care. So where should you start? The pointers below will help you build a top-notch Go To Team.

Follow Bloggers Who Know Their Stuff

There's a revolution going on in black hair care and it *is* being televised...on YouTube that is. I love YouTube! Even now, I can spend hours at a time watching videos about natural hair.

When I first started transitioning, my hair mentor Deanie directed me to bloggers and regularly sent me emails with tips about natural hair care. But soon, I was off and running on my own. I devoured information on natural hair and spent hours every week following my favorite bloggers and searching for new ones. I often sat in bed late into the night watching one YouTube video after another on my iPad, taking notes on product suggestions.

The success of my natural hair journey is due in large part to the host of YouTube bloggers who publicly shared their knowledge and hair care tips. I learned almost everything I know about the care of my hair from my sister bloggers. I am so grateful for the community of women who are graciously sharing their knowledge with the masses.

I encourage you to identify experienced bloggers you like and subscribe to their websites or YouTube channels. I love checking my email and finding out that one of my favs has posted a new article or video. Whether you become as addicted as I am or only check in every now and then, you'll learn a lot.

Here are some tips for selecting a blogger to guide you in your natural hair education.

Look for Hugely Popular Bloggers
Find a blogger with loads of subscribers (like thousands or hundreds of thousands). That's a sign of their popularity and an indication that they're imparting great hair care knowledge that people are clamoring to hear.

Find a Blogger with a Hair Type Similar to Yours
Find at least three experienced bloggers whose hair type appears similar to yours. That will give you a sense of whether the products they use might also work for you. *However, don't rule out following a blogger solely because she has a different hair texture.* Doing that means that you may be missing out on some great

information. One of my favorite bloggers is Mahogany Curls. My hair texture and curl pattern is nothing like hers. I follow her, however, because she offers invaluable hair care advice.

Find a Blogger Who Posts Regularly

Find a blogger who posts new videos a minimum of two or three times a month. That tells you that blogging is more than just a pastime for her. Her frequency in posting videos means she's committed to educating others and is keeping abreast of what's going on in the natural hair care world.

Don't Rule Out a Blogger Simply Because She Straightens Her Hair

Don't rule out a blogger simply because she isn't natural. A relaxed blogger, Hairlista, got me started on my journey. She is extremely knowledgeable about hair care and the information on her website is fantastic. Without her hair care advice, I might not be where I am today.

Find a Blogger Who Has Documented Her Journey in Pictures

If you can, find a blogger who has also gone through the natural hair process from a relaxer or a TWA, and has the photographs to prove it. Many of the bloggers I follow went from teeny weeny afros to long, gorgeous manes and they've documented their journeys on YouTube. Those are the bloggers who motivate me the most. If they can do it, so can you!

Browse YouTube for Topics of Interest

You may also want to peruse YouTube and discover a few bloggers on your own. I've listed several popular natural hair search terms to get you started. If you have a particular product you're interested in, search for the product name along with the word "review" or "tutorial".

co-washing	natural hair journey
going natural	shingling natural hair
natural hair	transitioning
natural hair types	twist out
pre-pooing	wash 'n go
retaining length	natural hair tutorial
natural hair products	deep conditioning

Pick Your Bloggers Carefully

There are no requirements for becoming a YouTube blogger. You just sign up for your free channel and start yapping. That said, everybody on YouTube doesn't warrant being followed. In my early days, I would follow the advice of anybody *claimed* that a product worked. I'm quite embarrassed now to admit some of the stuff my desperate self ran out and did. (Like buying a product made for horses' manes or putting Monistat 7—yes, the yeast infection remedy—on my scalp. I was desperate, y'all!)

Oddly enough, you'll also find quite a few bloggers on YouTube with hair that is tore up from the floor up.

When I look at the hair of some of those bloggers, all I can do is shake my head. Them trying to impart natural hair knowledge would've been like me posting those chicken head pictures on page 12 on YouTube and announcing to the world: "Hey, follow me. I'm going to help you grow healthy natural hair." What makes my voice one you might want to listen to now is that I've transformed my hair from a disastrous state to strong and healthy. In my mind, that alone says I must have attained some knowledge along the way. So set high expectations for the bloggers you follow!

Pamela's Best Bloggers List

I've listed below my Top 12 Favorite Bloggers. There are others I follow from time to time as well, but these sisters are my go-to girls for the reasons set forth below. You'll need to do your own research to find the bloggers you want to adopt as your hair mentors. There are a multitude of them out there!

To locate the bloggers mentioned below, visit their website or simply type in their name in the YouTube search box. To find a particular video that I've referenced, type the blogger's name and the title of the video in the YouTube search box.

CurlyNikki (YouTube)
CurlyNikki.com

Curly Nikki's website is as close as you'll get to natural hair college. The site offers visitors a collection of articles and videos from other bloggers, which means it's not just one blogger's viewpoint, but a variety of opinions and recommendations. The articles are always well-written, relevant and informative. If you want to know *anything* about your natural hair, you're likely to find it at CurlyNikki.com. I urge you to subscribe to CurlyNikki.com so that whenever new articles are posted, they will be sent to you via email.

UrbanBushBabes (YouTube)
UrbanBushBabes.com

Urban Bush Babes are two women who are definitely experts on growing natural hair. Talk about some hair! Take a look at theirs! These two sisters know how to make it grow! They offer fantastic tips on caring for your natural hair and retaining length. Be sure to check out their video series, *How to Grow Long Natural Hair.* Their website also covers style, arts & culture.

MahoganyCurls (YouTube)
Mahogany CurlsOnline.com

Mahogany Curls knows her stuff. Her tutorials are always well done and she doesn't waste your time with a lot of unnecessary chatter and fluff. It was amazing to watch her growth from a TWA to the most incredibly fabulous natural curls. Make sure you check out her video, *Big Chop: 1 Year Natural* and compare how far she's come since her teeny weeny afro days. As of the writing of this book, Mahogany Curls has nearly 200,000 subscribers.

Naptural85 (YouTube)
Naptural85.com

Naptural85 is another extremely knowledgeable blogger I simply adore! If you want some innovative ways for styling your hair, this is the place to go. Naptural85 also has some of the best hair product recipes ever. She has over 400,000 subscribers and has posted nearly 170 videos. Follow her and you'll learn a lot.

Kimmaytube (YouTube)
LoveNaturals.com

KimmayTube is committed to educating her subscribers. It's been amazing to see her tremendous hair growth documented on YouTube. I'm so glad that she's sharing her knowledge with the world. Definitely check out her YouTube videos on hair porosity and pH balance. She breaks it down like a college professor. KimmayTube even has her own product line, Luv Naturals. I love her headbands and styling products. You go girl!

BlackOnyx77 (YouTube)
Blackonyxworld.com

I can't wait until the day that my hair is long enough to sport a twist out like this sister's! She rocks in terms of her product reviews, tutorials and overall hair advice. Her YouTube videos have close to 12 million views! Her site includes not just hair advice, but fashion, makeup and other beauty tips too!

SimplYounique (YouTube)

This is another sister whose hair tips and advice helped me tremendously in reaching my natural hair goals. She was one of the first bloggers I began to follow. You *must* check out SimplYounique's video, *How I Grew My Natural Hair, Length Retention.* It will make you a believer.

Hairlicious, Inc. (YouTube)
Hairlista.com

You never forget your first. I discovered Hairlista at the beginning of my journey when I was desperately trying to grow out my relaxer. Her video, *My Hair Care Journey*, was the first YouTube hair video I ever watched. I encourage you to watch it too. As of the writing of this book, that video had nearly 650,000 views. I was floored by her long, beautiful permed hair (don't hate!) that she grew all by her lonesome. I was even more impressed by the wealth of knowledge on her website.

MyNaturalSistas (YouTube)

With over 200,000 subscribers, bloggers My Natural Sistas are definitely imparting some knowledge. What makes their blog unique is that it offers natural hair care advice from three different bloggers who just happen to be sisters. In addition to sharing their natural hair wisdom, they offer tips on makeup, health, fashion and more. Be sure to check out one of my favorite Natural Sistas videos, *How to Define Natural Curls for Kinky Curly Hair Tutorial.*

AfricanExport (YouTube)
AfricanExportBlog.com

I love African Export because she tells it like it is. She rocks her hair both natural and straight (don't hate!) and is crazy knowledgeable. I've learned a great deal from her, especially about conditioning my natural hair. She's posted over 900 videos. She also wears her hair in incredibly versatile styles. Check out one of my favorite deep conditioning recipes presented in African Export's video, *Natural Hair Talk + My Natural Hair Secret Weapon for Moisture.*

CharyJay (YouTube)
Chary-Jay.com

CharyJay is another fabulous blogger with natural hair to die for. Her videos are informative, well done and creative. If you're searching for ideas for great natural hairstyles, this is the place to go. If you can't find a style here, it doesn't exist. Check out her fantastic product reviews and makeup tips too.

Black Girl Long Hair
BlackGirlLongHair.com

This website is another place that I regularly turn to for informative articles on natural hair care. The site is well-organized and the photographs are fabulous. Like Curly Nikki's site, you'll find a variety of naturals sharing their advice on BlackGirlLongHair.com.

Two Bonus Bloggers

ColouredBeautiful (YouTube)
ColouredBeautiful.com

This sister is beautiful, talented and all-around fabulous. No single blogger has been more influential in my natural hair journey. She introduced me to the Mommy Wig and Kinky Curly Curling Custard. Both of those products saved me during my early transitioning period. She's also a fantastic makeup artist and trendsetter. I've watched her makeup tutorials over and over again. Be sure to check out one of my favorite Coloured Beautiful videos: *Natural Hair Rollercoaster.*

Kinky Coily Pamela (YouTube)
PamelaSamuelsYoung.com
Meetup.com/Natural-Born-Beauties

Yes, you'll also find me on YouTube. I don't have thousands of followers (yet!), but I'm working on it. So check me out and please subscribe! You'll also find a few hair tips and excerpts of my mystery novels on my website. If you're in the L.A. area, please join my Meetup group, Natural Born Beauties, and let's meet in person!

Many of these bloggers can also be found on Facebook and Instagram. If you're a blogger, please don't hate me for not including your blog. It would be impossible for me to include everyone. For an additional list of bloggers you may want to follow, see the list on page 142.

Participate in Online Forums

You can also enhance your learning curve by subscribing to online forums. There are many forums where you can post your questions and get responses from other naturals. You can also check the message boards to see if your question has already been posed by another natural. Here are a few to try out.

- **Long Hair Care Forum**
  longhaircareforum.com

- **Black Hair Media**
  forum.blackhairmedia.com

- **NapturallyCurly.com**
  napturallycurly.com/forums

Devour Books and Magazines on Natural Hair Care

I'm a writer as well as a voracious reader. So in addition to following my sister bloggers in my search for hair help, I also sought out books on natural hair. Here are my Top 10 picks. You'll find a more comprehensive list of books on natural hair on page 143.

Recommended Books
About Natural Hair Care

The Science of Black Hair: A Comprehensive Guide to Textured Hair Care by Audrey Davis-Sivasothy.

This was the first book that caught my eye when I began my search on Amazon for books on natural hair care. The book turned out to be a Godsend and has since become my natural hair Bible. If you're a kinky-textured woman who wants to *really* understand your hair, this is the book to read. I'll even go as far to say that if you can only afford one book, don't buy mine. Buy Audreys! (Yeah, I know, you already bought it.) *The Science of Black Hair* is essentially an encyclopedia on textured hair. The author is a health scientist and long-time, healthy hair care advocate. She writes extensively on the intricacies of caring for hair at home.

Better Than Good Hair: The Curly Girl Guide to Healthy, Gorgeous Natural Hair! by Nikki Walton and Ernessa T. Carter.

If you've been paying close attention, you already know that Nikki Walton, aka Curly Nikki, is one of my favorite natural hair bloggers. So I don't sound like a groupie or crazed stalker, I won't go on and on about her book. Just take my word for it that her advice is solid and her recipes and product recommendations are fabulous. As I've said earlier, Curly Nikki's website has a wealth of information on kinky hair, so you know her book is da bomb. Nuf said.

Natural Care for Curls and Kinks by Todra Payne.
This book is another must-read! The author is a celebrity makeup artist and the creator of HealthyBeautyProject. com, a site that provides information on the latest trends in natural and organic cosmetics. Her book teaches readers how to care for kinky-textured hair with natural and organic products. I loved the recipes (be sure to try the hair detox recipe), the advice on using essential oils and the options for natural hair coloring. You'll also find live links to recommended reading, product recommendations and links to YouTube videos.

If You Love It, It Will Grow: A Guide to Healthy, Beautiful Natural Hair by Phoenyx Austin.
The author of this book is a physician, author and entrepreneur who regularly blogs on fitness and women's lifestyle topics. Her book is chock full of helpful information which is delivered with the authority of a medical professional. She goes to great lengths to help readers understand the science of the hair. The author's own gorgeous tresses, which are featured on the cover of the book, tell me Dr. Austin knows what she's talking about.

Textured Tresses: The Ultimate Guide to Maintaining and Styling Natural Hair by Diane Da Costa with Paula Renfroe.
Diane Da Costa is a hair stylist to the stars who knows her stuff. Released in 2004, before the explosion of interest in natural hair among African-American women,

the book is still relevant today. Diane was helping her clients twist, braid and loc long before it became the *in* thing to do. You'll definitely learn a few things from this fantastic book.

Curly Girl: The Handbook by Lorraine Massey.
While not specifically written for African-American women, this book was the first of its kind for curly, textured hair. The author is the owner of the famed Devachan Salon in New York City. She does commit a chapter to us girls with kinky curls and, for me, her explanation of curl types was the first time that I really *got it* and was able to identify my curl pattern.

Get Your Length! Helping Women with Natural Hair Retain Length by Sais Sharpe and Anthony Policastro.
This book provides readers with the history of hair care within the African diaspora and is also a social study and memoir. It provides tips on retaining length with simple, easy-to-follow instructions. The author also takes us along on her natural hair journey and shares her personal hair regimen.

Milady Standard: Natural Hair Care and Braiding by Diane Carol Bailey and Diane Da Costa
Milady is the number one provider of educational resources for cosmetology schools around the world. This book on natural hair care is intended for stylists, so you know that it covers the gamut. It includes step-by-step

photos and detailed instructions for caring for natural hair. Milady promotes the book as a "must have for those who are serious about developing a wide range of services and building a broad, diverse client base."

Hair Care Rehab: The Ultimate Hair Repair & Reconditioning Manual by Audrey Davis-Sivasothy.
If you haven't caught on yet, I'm a big fan of Audrey Davis-Sivasothy, the author of *The Science of Black Hair.* Her second book, *Hair Care Rehab,* is just as fantastic as her first. This is another one of my go-to books, particularly if there's a hair care problem I'm trying to solve.

Natural Hair for Young Women by Phylecia Tarael-ANU, Aimè Tudor-ANU (Editor), H. Yuya Assaan-ANU (Editor).
Don't let the title fool you. This book has something for everyone, young, old and in-between. The author and editors went to great lengths to research natural hair and the results are fabulous. What I like most is their holistic approach to natural hair, which is aimed at teaching young girls to appreciate their God-given textures and helping them understand that they don't have to conform to supposed standards of beauty that do not apply to them.

There are lots of other great books out there and still more are hitting the market every day. You'll find a list of additional books on natural hair on page 143.

Natural Hair Care Magazines

It saddens me that as of the writing of this book, the major black hair magazines have not yet fully embraced the natural hair revolution. You'll find an article here and there on natural hair, but our pressed, permed and weaved sisters still dominate the pages of these publications. (I ain't hatin'. I just want some magazine space for us kinky coily girls!). With the explosion of interest in natural hair, I suspect we'll see more natural hair magazines hitting the market soon. By the way, have you noticed the growing predominance of kinky-textured sisters in television commercials and print advertising? It makes me proud!

The magazines below are spreading the word. Please support them and subscribe!

Naptural Roots

napturalroots.com

When I browse through the photos of all the beautiful women in this magazine, I am so proud to be natural! Available in both digital and print, *Naptural Roots*, started as a way to give a voice to the growing natural hair community. *Naptural Roots* now covers not just hair care, but skin care, health and fitness, wellness, spirituality and more.

The Coil Review

thecoilreview.com

Billed as a natural hair web magazine, The *Coil Review* is all about natural hair. It has great articles on a wide range of topics relevant to naturals. You should definitely check out the *New Natural, Regimen* and *Recipe* sections. There's surely something there to help you with your journey. Their photo pages are stunning and a great place to find some new styling options.

Naturally Happy Hair

naturallyhappyhair.com

Naturally Happy Hair magazine is a national print and digital magazine that provides resources on styling, hair care and products for all natural hair types. You'll also find articles on the natural lifestyle, events and members of the natural hair community.

Natura

naturamagazineusa.com

Natura magazine was created with the goal of inspiring and changing the ideals of beauty among women of color. The magazine bills itself as a "celebration of natural hair, skin, and the true essence of a woman of color." Says the creator of *Natura*: "My main goal for *Natura* is to create a platform for women to express themselves, and be confident about their natural hair, skin, and beauty. I know the importance of hair to a woman, and I wanted to create a magazine that not only publicized natural hair, but also inspired women to rock it with confidence."

Mhe

mhemagazine.com

Mhe (My hair experience) is a beauty-centric consumer-focused magazine dedicated to providing inspiration for the modern day woman who has chosen to rock her natural hair. The vision for the magazine is that every woman reading it will see herself through its pages and be able to both benefit from the styles and information provided and contribute by sharing her individual journey. The magazine provides an abundance of resources, tips, product reviews, how-to tutorials, style pictures and a where-to directory that showcases local salons, empowering women everywhere with options on how to care for and maintain their natural hair texture.

Natural Style
naturalstylemagazine.com
Natural Style is a magazine dedicated exclusively to the natural hair and loc-wearing community. It provides a comprehensive source for the latest trends, techniques and tips to those who are natural or in transition. The magazine partners with top natural stylists, natural product developers and members of the natural hair wearing community to create a thorough and creative publication.

Natural Hollywood
naturalhollywood.com
Natural Hollywood provides exclusive access to everything fabulous, trendy and hot about natural hair. All of the models featured in the magazine demonstrate a unique personality while rocking an exclusive natural hair creation by the owner and stylist of Naturally Me, Jennifer Lord.

Midwest Black Hair

midwestblackhair.com

Midwest Black Hair is a monthly publication devoted to showcasing African-American hair styles, promoting local hair and beauty stylists, supporting local small businesses, putting a spotlight on hair & beauty events in the Midwest, and providing hair, beauty, and health information specifically for people of color.

Connect with Other Naturals

Some of my best hair care tips and product recommendations have come from other naturals. Itr's important to surround yourself with other women who are as excited as you are about going natural. Why do you need other naturals? For encouragement, information and support. I've found some of my favorite products (Uncle Funky's Daughter Curly Magic!) as a result of a tip from another natural. There will be times when you need the support because some of our unenlightened family, friends and co-workers just don't get it. They tend to be more comfortable with your straight hair and they won't understand why you'd want to go natural. But as long as *you* appreciate your hair, that's the most important thing. And something amazing is going to happen, once they see you rocking your kinky coils, people you thought would never go natural, will follow right behind you. Here are a few suggestions for connecting with other naturals.

Join Natural Hair Groups

I'm proud to be part of a community of women who enjoy talking hair. Meetup.com, the social networking site that allows members to connect with others who share a common interest, is a great way to meet other naturals. Just do a search on Meetup.com for natural hair groups in your area. Whether you decide to join a formal group or just chat with other friends or family members who have gone natural, you'll benefit from the exchange. If you can't find any groups in your area, you'll find a ton of online forums.

I've attended product swaps and gatherings to discuss natural hair. It's quite motivating to be in a room full of beautiful natural women. You can also start your own group. In fact, I've formed a Meetup group of my own, Natural Born Beauties.

Attend Conferences and Workshops

I'm happy to see more and more natural hair conferences popping up. So many that there are far too many of them to list here. Isn't that fabulous? To find out what conferences are planned for your area, search your city and "natural hair shows" on Google. Or, you can visit, MyNaturalHairEvents.com.

My Natural Hair Events
www.mynaturalhairevents.com
My Natural Hair Events provides the latest information on hair events around the globe, from large natural hair shows and expos to small neighborhood

Meetup groups, as well as natural hair workshops and seminars. So check out the site to see what's happening in your town. You can even submit your own event for posting on the site.

Make New Natural Friends Everywhere

I can't tell you how many naturals I've connected with in the grocery store line, in department stores and at parties. When I see another natural whose hair I admire, I don't hesitate to say so and that *always* leads to a discussion about products and/or hairstyles. There is a growing community of new naturals where I work and I've watched many of my personal friends transition to natural hair too. I have girlfriends who I thought would *never* go natural, but now they're giving it a try. Share the wealth, meet a natural!

Create Your Personal Go To Team

You are likely to run into roadblocks along the way and will need to consult with a natural who's more experienced than you are. So it's important to have a Go To Team. Use the resources above to create one.

Make a list of the following:

- Your favorite bloggers and forums.

- Natural hair books you want to read and magazines you want to subscribe to.

- Natural hair groups you want to join and conferences you plan to attend.

- Your new natural friends.

- Your natural hair professional.

It's also great to have a natural hair mentor, some-one who's been natural far longer than you and who can calm you down when you run into a little hair drama.

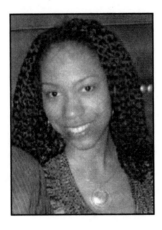

My mentor, Latrice Byrdsong, is the twist-out queen and rocks some very creative protective styles. She is also incredibly knowledgeable about natural hair care and products.

So start looking. Potential mentors are all around you. Your Go To Team won't be complete without one.

STEP THREE
Design Your Personal Natural Hair Care Regimen

Taking the first step in designing your personal natural hair care regimen can seem daunting. There are so many products, so many processes and, in the early stages of your journey, a lack of knowledge about your hair's precise needs. My advice? Don't fret over designing the perfect routine. Just get started. My routine changes every six months or so. I either add a product or take one away. It's going to take some trial and error to find the products that work best for you. I recommend that before you create your regimen, spend some time sopping up a little knowledge from your Go To Team (natural bloggers, books, magazines, friends, etc.). They may be able to help you avoid some costly mistakes.

When I started my natural hair journey, the more I learned, the more amazed I was at all the things I *didn't* know about my hair. They're obviously not teaching this stuff in cosmetology school, because I've even had hair stylists ask *me* for hair advice and product tips.

About six months into my journey, I became quite saddened by the fact that I'd spent most of my life being dissatisfied with my hair, having no idea that I had a natural curl pattern. Growing up, I longed for *good* hair. I realize now that what I have is much better than good hair. It's *great* hair. That's why I'm so excited about sharing my natural hair knowledge with other women.

Before you can create a regimen that works for you, you will need to evaluate the current condition of your hair. Can you plunge in right away or will you need to do the big chop? The next section will help you answer that question.

To Chop or Not to Chop

If your hair is relaxed or damaged, deciding whether to take the plunge and do the big chop is one of the most difficult decisions you will have to make as you begin your natural hair journey.

When I started my transition, I was determined that I would *not* do the big chop. I wanted length and I was determined to keep what little thin, damaged, scraggily hair I had left. I also didn't want to wear a TWA (teeny weeny afro). I was convinced that I wouldn't look good with short hair. My inability to find a suitable hairstyle during the early part of my transitioning process was quite frustrating. My hair was too short to simply pull back in a ponytail. Sometimes I slicked it back with gel (which was drying), but my edges were nearly bald, so that wasn't much of a solution. My hair was in such an awful state that the best transitioning option for me was hiding my damaged hair underneath a wig.

Months later, I gathered the courage to do the big chop. And only then—after cutting off my perm-damaged hair—did my hair begin to flourish.

Here are a few pros and cons to consider as you ponder your decision about the big chop.

You Should Consider the Big Chop if . . .

1   You're impatient and ready to rock your natural hair now!
2   You love the ideal of a short hairdo.
3   Your hair is severely damaged.
4   You're not ready for all the work required by a transitioning regimen.
5   Spending months growing out your relaxer will drive you batty.

You Should Not Consider the Big Chop if . . .

1   You don't want to wear a TWA (teeny, weeny afro).
2   You don't think you'll look good in short hair.
3   Your hair is fairly healthy and you don't want to lose your length.
4   You're patient enough to wait months or years to grow out your relaxed hair.
5   You don't mind putting in the work required to transition to natural hair.

What to Do with Your Hair During Your Transition if the Big Chop Isn't for You

One reason many women decide not to transition to natural hair is because they can't find a satisfactory way to wear their hair during the transitioning process. That's definitely how I felt. I've listed a few options below.

Buns
This is an option if you have sufficient length. A bun is also considered a protective hairstyle because your ends are tucked in and not exposed.

Wigs
There are some great wigs out there that look very natural. Even some of my closest friends thought my Mommy wig was my real hair. They thought I'd gotten a cute new haircut. Wearing a wig is a perfectly reasonable option for many women. You can even find wigs that look like twist-outs. My friend Shar gets stopped all the time for natural hair tips because her kinky-textured wig looks so marvelous. She rarely tells people it's not her hair. She just passes on some of the natural hair tips I've given her and tells them about my book. LOL! Check out my tutorial on the Mommy wig, which I wore during my transitioning process, on my YouTube Channel Kinky Coily Pamela.

Weaves
Many women choose to wear a weave during the transitioning process. Just make sure your braids are not too tight and that the weave isn't damaging your hair.

Cornrows
Cornrows are another low-stress hairstyle that will allow your hair to grow, provided they're not too tight.

Braids
Long before I decided to go natural, I wore braids for three years and my hair grew fabulously during that period. Just make sure you properly care for your braids and that they aren't too tight, particularly around the delicate edges. Check out Naptural85 on on YouTube and the book *Going Natural: How to Fall in Love with Nappy Hair* by Mireille Liong-a-kong for some braided hair styling ideas.

Whether you transition to natural hair by slowly growing out your relaxed hair or go for the big chop is a personal decision only *you* can make.

Developing A Natural Hair Care Regimen
As I've said repeatedly, natural hair care can be very time intensive, which is why having a specific regimen to follow is advised. Your regimen must take into account your hair type and curl pattern and what they require, the amount of time you can devote to your hair care on a weekly or daily basis, the condition of your hair and your specific hair goals. Your weekly regimen should include when you plan to wash (or co-wash), deep condition and moisturize and seal. Your regimen should also note when plan to trim, color or do protein treatments.

The Products You'll Need to Get Started

At a minimum, you'll need the following products as you commence your natural hair journey.

- Co-wash/Shampoo (sulfate-free)
- Leave-in Conditioner
- Deep Conditioner
- Moisturizer
- Curl Definer (gel or cream)
- Oils and Butters
- Water!
- Wide-tooth comb
- Plastic caps
- Heat cap

How Much Time Can You Commit?

One of my friends has beautiful, long thick hair. But nobody knew it because she always wears a wig. When she finally announced that she was going natural, I was thrilled. She showed me a lock of her hair and I was stunned that she was hiding that gorgeous hair underneath a wig! I gave her lots of tips and the next time I saw her she was rocking a twist-out I would kill for. Several friends also raved about how great her hair looked.

Her natural hairdo, however, didn't last for long. A few weeks later I ran into her and she was sporting another weave.

"What happened?" I asked.

"Girl, that took too much work."

"It gets easier over time," I said, but she wasn't hearing it.

Is that you? How much time can you commit?

You wouldn't start a diet without a routine, would you? Well, don't start your natural hair journey without a plan. Your hair care regimen is your roadmap to natural hair. What you do and how you do it will depend on your hair and your hair goals. So do your homework and find out what works for you. To give you an idea of what a regimen looks like, here's a look at my initial regimen and my current regimen.

Sample Natural Hair Care Regimens

Pamela's First Regimen

First, don't let my regimen overwhelm you. Depending on the condition of your hair, you don't have to be this intense. If you look back at the photographs on page 12, you should completely understand why I jumped into my natural hair journey with such passion. My hair was in horrendous shape and I was desperate to rescue it.

Co-wash: Monday, Wednesday and Saturday Mornings

I chose to wash my hair frequently, first because my hair tends to be very dry and I felt the water was good for my hair, and second because I used gels to shingle my hair which caused a lot of product buildup. You may want to cleanse your hair less frequently. That will depend on *your* hair's needs. I typically co-washed my hair using Herbal Essence Hello Hydration Conditioner. On some days, I co-washed with Wen Cleansing Conditioner, which I love, but don't use regularly despite loving the results because it's darn expensive when compared to the cost of other conditioners and co-washes.

I also washed in the morning because I didn't want to go to bed with wet hair and I like to have my hair fresh for the start of the day.

At least once a week after co-washing, I applied an apple cider vinegar rinse to clarify my hair because of my heavy use of gels to define my curls. You can find my Apple Cider Vinegar Clarifying Rinse recipe on page 132.

Moisturize and Seal: Nightly

Every night before I went to bed (unless I was feeling lazy), I used the LOC (liquid, oil, cream) method to moisturize and seal my hair. For my liquid, I used Luster's S Curl No Drip Curl Activator Moisturizer (yes the same one from back in the Jheri Curl days!) I then applied jojoba oil and topped it off with a cream. I used either Hollywood Beauty's Olive Oil Cream or Organic Roots Stimulator Olive Oil Incredibly Rich Moisturizing Hair Lotion.

At least once a week, I would bag my ends for added moisture. Make sure you're not heavy handed with the products. If you wake up the next morning and your hair is a greasy mess, use less product next time. By the way, I don't tie up my hair at night because I don't want to squash my curls. Instead I sleep on a satin pillowcase and it works out just fine.

Shingle Styling: After Every Co-Wash

After co-washing, I shingled my hair, which is the style on the cover of this book. To shingle my hair, I section off my hair with clips in 8 separate parts. I then applied Kinky Curly Curling Custard to a small section and twirled it around my finger. In the beginning this process took about an hour. Nowadays, it takes me 30-40 minutes. *Warning: This is not a protective or low-manipulation hairstyle*! And yes, I often left the house with my hair not fully dry. It takes about four hours for my hair to dry. Because I live in a warm climate (Los Angeles) going out into the elements with slightly damp hair hasn't been a problem for me.

Deep Condition: Sunday Night/Friday Night

I love my deep conditioning time! My first deep conditioning process included applying a special oil mixture (*see* page 133 for the recipe) to my scalp and hair along with either my homemade Shea Butter Mix (*see* page 133 for the recipe) or a deep conditioner such as Cantu Shea Butter Leave In Conditioning Cream or Organic Roots Stimulator's Hair Mayonnaise. I sat for at least an hour, sometimes two, under a heat cap. During that time I was either reading my hair Bible, *The Science of Black Hair,* surfing natural hair blogs or watching YouTube videos. (Yes, I am quite the fanatic.)

Protein Treatment: Every 8 Weeks
Hair needs protein for strength. I love Aphogee Two Step Protein Treatment. After applying this product, I sat under a hooded hairdryer (not a heat cap). Don't be alarmed when your hair becomes hard. That's intended. Read the instructions on the bottle and follow them carefully.

Covering My Gray
As discussed earlier, I have gray primarily along my hairline, which I cover every four to five weeks. I use either henna with indigo powder or Deity America Color Change Shampoo, which is plant-based.

Pamela's Current Hair Care Regimen

My current hair care regimen is not the same as my regimen when I first started my transition. For instance, I no longer bag my ends. I really benefited from this process when my hair was severely damaged, but now that it's healthier, I forgo this process. I've added steam treatments to my regimen and I don't wash my hair as frequently. The biggest change in my hair regimen is that I rarely co-wash these days. This change happened totally by accident. I was on a business trip without my conditioner and was forced to use shampoo. When I shingled my hair and applied my gel, I immediately noticed that my curls were shiny and more defined. I had not been using the apple cider vinegar rinse to clarify my hair after co-washing for some time.

This experience caused me to realize that conditioner alone wasn't cleansing the gel from my hair as well as shampoo did.

Wash: Every 3 to 4 Days

I went from co-washing my hair three times a week to washing it with a sulfate-free shampoo about twice a week. Over time, I began to notice that my curls stayed defined for a longer period of time without getting frizzy. Therefore, I didn't need to redo it so often. Since I use a curl defining gel to shingle my hair after every wash, I now prefer a co-wash product or a sulfate-free shampoo to cleanse my hair rather than conditioner. I can honestly say that these products do a better job of removing the gel from my hair. I still co-wash with one of the many Herbal Essence conditioners when I'm giving my hair a break from shingling.

Styling: Shingle Hair After Every Wash

I still shingle my hair and love that style. As noted earlier, this is not a protective or low-manipulation style. I've never worn protective styles because my hair isn't long enough to pull into a bun and I didn't want to wear cornrows or other braided styles. Why have hair you love if you can't wear it out? So I deliberately made the decision not to wear a protective/low-manipulation style because I love the kinky coily look and the tradeoff (less length retention) works just fine for me.

Moisturize and Seal: When Needed

I no longer use the LOC method (liquid, oil, cream) every night. Now I LOC only when needed, which is more like once or twice a week. On almost a daily basis, however, I will spritz my hair with water when I get home from work. When my hair feels dry, I'll spritz it with Luster S Curl No Drip Curl Activator Moisturizer or apply my favorite cream, As I Am Double Butter Cream, before going to bed.

Deep Condition: Once a Week

I now only deep condition once a week rather than twice a week. I've recently started using Camille Rose Naturals Algae Renew Deep Conditioner. My favorite deep conditioning oils these days are Taliah Waajid's Black Earth African Healing Oyl and Treasured Locks African Argan Elixir. I still use my time under the heat cap to continue my hair care education by surfing natural hair blogs or watching YouTube videos.

Steam Treatment: Once a Month

Steaming my hair is one of my special hair treats. I purchased a hair steamer on Amazon.com and I love it. My normally coarse hair becomes soft and moisturized after just 10 or 15 minutes under my steamer. I will sometimes combine my steam treatment with my deep conditioning treatment.

Protein treatment: Every 10-12 Weeks

My protein treatments are also less frequent these days, every 10 to 12 weeks, rather than every 8 weeks.

Hair Detox: Every 8 to 10 Weeks

Every 8 to 10 weeks or so, I detox my hair using Terressentials Pure Earth Hair Wash (either the Lemon or Lavender Garden). This is a clay-like cleanser that really clarifies my hair. As soon as I apply it, my curls jump to attention. I love this product and my hair loves it too.

Every 3 Months: Trim or Dusting

In the beginning of my journey, I did not trim my hair because I wanted to retain every bit of length I had, even though it wasn't worth saving.

Have you ever gone in for a trim and ended up with your stylist cutting off way more hair than you expected? I have. For that reason, I was reluctant to put my hair in the hands of a stylist armed with a pair of scissors. Although I went to a stylist I trust for my big chop, I now do my own trimmings, which are really more like dustings, because I trim very little hair, just the scraggily ends. So far, this works for me. You must decide if you want to do the same or go to a professional stylist for a trim. Just find one that you trust.

Hopefully, my regimen didn't scare you off. It might sound like a lot of work, but anything worth having takes effort. The time I spend caring for my natural hair is far less than the hour I spent driving to the beauty salon (one way) and sitting for a perm, color or a weave. More importantly, I also have the satisfaction of knowing that I'm in charge of my own hair care. For me, that's empowering.

Now that you're ready to begin your journey, it's important to put your plan in writing.

Journal About Your Natural Hair Journey

If you're serious about your journey, you'll need a journal. You can purchase the *Kinky Coily Natural Hair Journal* or use the information below to create your own journal. If you plan to do the latter, I recommend using a small, three-ring binder that will allow you to add sheets.

Don't stress over creating the perfect natural hair care regimen. It doesn't (and shouldn't) be set in stone. Your regimen will change as your natural hair knowledge grows, as your hair changes, and as you discover new and more effective products.

At a minimum, your journal should include the elements listed below.

- **What are your natural hair goals?**
- **Are you...**
  - Transitioning from a relaxer?
  - Doing the big chop?
  - Already natural?
- **Will you wash or co-wash?**
- **What protective styles will you wear?**

Products You'll Need to Purchase

- Shampoo/Co-wash
- Leave-in Conditioner
- Deep Conditioner
- Oils

- Gel
- Cream/Butter

Keep track of the following:

o Products you like (and why).

o Products you did not like (and why).

o Products you'd like to try.

o The Tools You'll Need

Here's a checklist of some of the tools you may want to have on hand.

- Wide-tooth comb
- Denman brush
- Plastic caps
- Hair clips
- Spray and tint bottles
- Plastic containers (for mixing products)
- Lint-free towel/old T-shirt
- Satin scarf/pillowcase
- Heat cap
- Blow dryer/diffuser
- Hooded dyer
- Steamer
- Latex gloves
- Afro pic

Your Natural Hair Care Schedule

Some people think keeping a schedule of what you do to your hair is overkill, but maintaining a regular schedule is important. Sometimes I couldn't remember whether I washed my hair yesterday or the day before. Having a written schedule will make it easier to keep track of your routine.

To keep track of your schedule, you can use the *Kinky Coily Natural Hair Journal*. If you want to create your own journal, I recommend printing out a free yearly calendar (in a monthly format) from the Internet and inserting it in a 3-ring binder.

Determine in advance how many times and what days of the week you plan do the following tasks, then schedule them in your journal.

- Wash/co-wash
- Deep condition
- Moisturize and seal
- Trim/dust
- Color
- Henna

Pamela's 10-Point Checklist for a Successful Natural Hair Journey

✓ Create Your Weekly Regimen.

✓ Keep Your Hair Clean and Moisturized.

✓ Deep Condition Weekly.

✓ Use Protective and Low-Manipulation Hairstyles.

✓ Stay Away from the Heat!

✓ Make Water Your BFF.

✓ Trim Your Ends When Needed.

✓ Take a Hair Vitamin Daily.

✓ Continue Your Natural Hair Education.

✓ Be Patient!

CHAPTER 4

Relax and Enjoy the Journey!

LOVE THE TITLE OF THE book by Curly Nikki and Ernessa T. Carter: *Better than Good Hair.* That's right. They said it and I'm saying it too. Our hair is *better* than *good* hair.

For me, going natural has been a liberating experience. I like the fact that I'm in charge of my hair care. I can ride in a convertible without the wind revealing my weave tracks and I can take a stroll in the rain without wrecking my hairstyle. In fact, my hair loves the rain!

During my early natural days, I stressed a lot. I stressed over my hair taking forever to grow. I stressed about finding the right style. I stressed over shrinkage. But soon, everything clicked and I hit my stride and found a pep in my step. Now that I'm natural, I can't imagine why it took me so long.

Final Thoughts

Here are some final thoughts I'd like you to keep in mind as you commence your natural hair journey.

Tweak What You've Learned to Fit Your Needs

I've said it before and I'm saying it this one last time. We all have different hair textures, therefore, what works for one natural may not work for another. As you read this book and as you gain knowledge about natural hair care from other sources, tweak it to fit your needs. Nothing I've written in this book is set in stone. Not even for me. My routine is constantly changing. Be discerning in your choice of bloggers to follow and products to buy. When you hear about a product or process you think you might like, don't be discouraged if it doesn't work out. Tweak it to fit your personal needs.

Ignore the Unenlightened

Now that I've gotten you all excited and revved up about going natural, I need to warn you that not everyone around you will be as excited as you are about your transition to natural hair. My mother loves my hair, but my father has yet to come around. When he saw my temporarily straight hair on New Year's Eve, he immediately told me how good I looked, then said: "You're not gonna nap it back up, are you?" I promptly assured him, that yes, I definitely planned to "nap it back up." LOL!

As far as my hair is concerned, if I'm happy with it, that's what counts most. That may or may not be the case for you. But if you transition to natural hair, you will have to realize that many, many people are not used to seeing your natural hair and are most comfortable with seeing you in a pressed or relaxed state.

But that's quickly changing. I'm spotting more and more glamorous naturals everywhere I turn. What you're going to find is that the women who turned up their noses when you first went natural, three or four months later will be asking you questions about transitioning. Heck, you were probably one of those women who turned up your nose.

My issue isn't that everyone should go natural, but that everyone should know what their hair *can* do. I've had frustrating discussions with women who insist that they do not have a curl pattern and no product in the world could make their hair curl. When I show them differently, they just stand there in front of the mirror with their mouths gaped open.

What I'm seeing in hair care among my kinky-textured sisters is nothing short of revolutionary. With the aid of the Internet, we're talking about our hair and freely sharing our resources. What's most interesting to me is that when I watch television commercials, I'm seeing far more natural sisters than not. The wig and weave shops better watch out. Their customer base is dwindling!

So hang in there when you come across the unenlightened. They just don't know what they're missing. In the words of Maya Angelou, "When you know better, you do better."

Put in the Work

There's no way around doing the work to find out what works for *your* hair.

My niece recently sent me a photograph and asked, "Could I do this with my hair if I go natural?" While I initially said *yes*, I realized that I couldn't definitively answer her question. Everyone's hair texture and curl patterns are different. You have to find the right product for *your* hair. As I ultimately advised her, whether she could rock that style would depend on her curl type and the products she used. That can only come about by doing the work to learn *your* hair. There's no way around it.

Don't Become a Straighter Hater

Just as some of our non-natural sisters may look down on us naturals, we need to be careful not to do the same to those who choose not to rock their natural hair. How you wear your hair is a very personal choice and natural hair isn't for everyone. Lots of women just don't want to dedicate the time. We're not better because we wear our natural hair. So I urge my natural sisters not to be straighter haters.

That said, don't be surprised if you see me rockin' straight hair again one day. Not for the long haul, but just for a change of pace.

Share the Knowledge!

If you're anything like me, you're going to be amazed at how quickly all of the information you're learning about natural hair sinks in and passion takes over. I like learning about my hair and I enjoy testing new products and browsing the aisles of the beauty supply store looking for new natural hair care lines. I encourage you to share the knowledge you're learning with your friends, colleagues and family members who have no idea what's hiding underneath their wigs and weaves. And please encourage your mothers and grandmothers to give natural hair a try. It isn't just for the young. I'm proof of that. You may find it hard to convince them to try wearing their natural hair, but once you start rockin' yours, I guarantee you others will follow.

Good luck and continue to embrace the natural you!

CHAPTER 5

Resources

Pamela's Favorite Things

L IKE OPRAH, I HAVE MY Favorite Things and I'm more than happy to share them with you. But remember...what works for my hair, may not work for yours. Continue to experiment, talk with friends and consult with the blogging world until you find *your* favorites.

Recipes

As I've said earlier, I don't have the time or the inclination to spend a lot of time concocting my own hair products. But there are a few things that I do mix myself and I'm happy to share them with you.

Judy's Homemade Shampoo
4 oz. Dr. Bronner's Pure Castille Soap
4 oz. distilled water
1 ½ tablespoons vegetable glycerin
1 ½ tablespoons (total) of extra virgin olive oil,
    grapeseed oil and sweet almond oil.
10 drops tea tree oil (antiseptic to keep shampoo
    fresh longer)
5 drops sage oil (for growth)
5 drops rosemary oil (for growth)

Combine the ingredients above in a small spray bottle and shake. Only make a small amount because it won't stay fresh long.

My friend Judy Brown shared this recipe with me. She's been natural for over a decade and not only is she a hair stylist, but she's also a former cosmetology instructor who's spreading the natural hair gospel.

Apple Cider Vinegar Clarifying Rinse
1 part apple cider vinegar
4 parts water

Because I use a gel to shingle my hair, product buildup is a big concern for me. Once a week when I was co-washing, I used an apple cider vinegar rinse to clarify my hair. I still clarify my from time to time to remove product buildup from my hair. When making the rinse, use a tint bottle with measuring lines so you use the proper ratio of vinegar to water. Douse your hair with the rinse after co-washing or washing, then wash it out and add your leave-in conditioner.

Shea Butter Hair and Body Potion
½ cup of shea butter
1 tablespoon of coconut oil
1 tablespoon of jojoba oil
1 tablespoon of castor oil
1 tablespoon of grape seed oil
5 drops of lavender oil

Combine the above ingredients in a high speed blender until the texture is smooth and creamy. I use this potion on my hair and body.

Deep Conditioner
1 egg
¼ cup of olive oil
1 cup of conditioner (your choice)

Combine the ingredients listed above in a plastic container and mix well. Use this as a deep conditioner for 30 minutes under a heat cap. Your hair will love it.

Pamela's Hot Oil Treatment
2 tablespoons of castor oil
2 tablespoons of olive oil
2 tablespoons of jojoba oil
2 tablespoons of grapeseed oil

5 drops of tea tree oil
5 drops of lavender or rosemary oil

Mix the oils listed above in a tint bottle and apply to your hair and scalp. I particularly love this treatment with a heat cap.

Pamela's Proven Fix for Thinning Edges
Organic Root Stimulator Temple Balm
Rosemary oil
Shea butter or castor oil

All my life, I've had thin edges. After I began to experience severe hair breakage from a relaxer and heat damage, my temples went from thin to bald. Just to prove that I'm not exaggerating, here's another look at my before and after pictures.

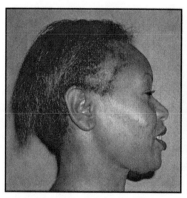 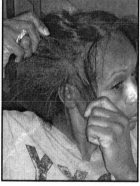

Once I began my natural hair education, I came to understand that because my kinky hair is so fragile, I needed to be more gentle with it, particularly around the edges. Here's the recipe and application technique that brought my edges back to life:

1. I massaged Organic Root Stimulator Temple Balm along my temples, morning and night. No need to be heavy handed. Just a little will do. Then I added a couple of drops of rosemary oil to my fingertips tips and massaged it into my temples. *Never apply rosemary oil directly to the scalp by itself! It's much too strong for direct contact and needs to be diffused with the temple balm.*

2. I made sure that my temples were properly moisturized *at all times.* If my edges looked or felt a little dry during the day, I would dab a little castor oil or shea butter (whichever I had handy) on them.

3. I also made sure that my temples were properly protected *at all times.* I avoided any type of head covering that would cause friction along my hairline. When I wore a baseball cap or even a wig, I sewed or taped a piece of satin fabric along the edge of the cap or wig to prevent friction. I slept on a satin pillowcase.

After about six weeks of the above treatment, I began to see peach fuzz in places that had previously been bald. In three months, I actually had enough hair to curl up with gel. By the six-month period, I actually had some length at my temples.

In the interest of full disclosure, I must reveal that I do have a couple of small spots along my temples where the hair did not grow back. Thankfully, there's enough hair in the areas to cover up those spots. Check out my video, *How I Repaired my Thinning Edges,* which you'll find on my YouTube channel, Kinky Coily Pamela.

Hair Products

Product choice is a very personal thing. What works for me, might not work for you. So it's important that you do your own research and experimentation. That said, here are a few of the products that I've personally used and that you might want to give a try.

Hair Cleansers (sulfate-free)

- Carol's Daughter Monoi (Repairing) Sulfate-free Shampoo *(My fav!)*

- Terraessentials Pure Earth Hair Wash *(Love it!)*

- Taliah Waajid Clean and Natural Herbal Hair Wash

- Tukka Cha'Cha All Natural Ultra Conditioning Sulfate-Free Shampoo

- Design Essentials Natural Curl Cleanser

- Hydratherma Naturals SLS Free Moisture Plus Hair Cleanser
- Curls Unleashed Organic Root Stimulator Lavish in Lather Sulfate-Free Shampoo
- Entwine Couture Cleansing & Growth Lathering Hair Bathè

Co-Washes

- Herbal Essence Hello Hydration & Hydralicious Conditioners
- Carol's Daughter Co-Wash Cleansing Conditioner
- Wen (Fig) Conditioning Cleanser by Chaz Dean
- As I Am Coconut Co-wash Cleansing Conditioner
- Sofn'free GroHealthy Nothing But Cleansing Conditioner

Leave-in Conditioners

- Kinky Curly Knot Today *(My fav!)*
- Blended Beauty Happy Nappy Styles Leave in Conditioner Butter
- Infusion 23 Conditioner
- Giovanni Hair Care Direct Leave in Conditioner
- Carol's Daughter Hair Milk Leave-in Moisturizer

- Profectiv Break Free Leave-in
- Curl Junkie Hibiscus & Banana Honey Butta Leave-In Conditioner
- Cantu Shea Butter Leave-in

Deep Conditioners

- Organic Roots Stimulator's Hair Mayonnaise
- Camille Rose Naturals Algae Renew Deep Conditioner.
- Cantu Shea Butter Grow Strong Conditioning Treatment
- Carol's Daughter Monoi Repairing Hair Mask *(One of my personal favorites! Also check out Carol's Daughter's Transitioning Kit.)*
- Elasta QP DPR-11+ Deep Penetrating Remoisturizing Conditioner
- Joico K-PAK RevitaLuxe Bio-Advanced Restorative Treatment
- Miss Jessie's Rapid Recovery Treatment
- Organic Root Stimulator Replenishing Pak
- Organic Root Stimulator Olive Oil Masque
- Tukka Natural Hair Care Treatment
- Carol's Daughter Olive Oil Infusion

Curl Definers

I've used a number of curl-enhancing gels and creams during my natural hair journey. Hands down, Uncle Funky's Daughter Curly Magic is my favorite. It's what I used when I styled my hair for the cover of this book. I like it because it's relatively light, doesn't flake or leave my hair dry and crunchy like some gels.

Here are some other popular curl-enhancing gels and creams that you may want to try out.

Gels

- Uncle Funky's Daughter Curly Magic (*My fav!*)
- Eco Styler Gel
- Fantasia ic Hair Polisher Styling Gel
- Kinky Curly Curling Custard
- Kiss My Face Upper Management Gel
- Organic Root Stimulator Curls Unleashed Curl Boosting Jelly

Creams

- As I Am Double Butter Cream *(My fav!)*
- Jane Carter Curl Defining Creme
- Miss Jessie's Baby Buttercream
- Hollywood Beauty Olive Oil Cream Hairdress for Dry Hair
- Entwine Couture Crème Jelle Styler

- Qhemet Biologics Amla & Heavy Cream
- Entwine Couture Crème De La Mode
- Curls Whipped Cream
- Qhemet Biologics Aethiopika Hydrate & Twist Butter

Moisturizers

- Organic Roots Stimulator Moisturizing Hair Lotion
- S Curl No Drip Activator Moisturizer
- Aphogee Balancing Moisturizer
- Tukka Koko Du Lait
- Entwine Couture Exotique Butter-Crème Hydrator

Oils

- Taliah Waajid Black Earth African Healing Oil
- Treasured Locks African Argan Elixir
- Qhemet Biologics Castor & Moringa Softening Serum

Products for Covering Gray Hair

- Diety America Color Change Shampoo
- Ancient Sunrise Henna for Gray Hair Kit

Protein Treatments

- Aphogee Two Step Protein Treatment
- Aphogee Keratin 2 Minute Reconstructor

Temple Balms

- Organic Root Stimulator Fertilizing Temple Balm
- Dr. Miracles Temple and Nape Gro Balm

Vitamins

- Hairfinity Hair Vitamins
- GNC Be Beautiful Hair, Skin and Nail (soft chews)

The following books offer extensive product recommendations. Please consult them to help you select the right products for your hair.

- *The Science of Black Hair: A Comprehensive Guide to Textured Hair Care* by Audrey Davis-Sivasothy, Chapter 7: Getting Started with a Healthy Hair Care Product Regimen.

- *Better Than Good Hair: The Curly Girl Guide to Healthy, Gorgeous Natural Hair!* by Nikki Walton and Ernessa T. Carter, Appendix, Your Natural Hair Product Guide.

- *Natural Care for Curls and Kinks* by Todra Payne.

Bloggers

I'm grateful for the many natural hair bloggers who are teaching women with kinky hair about the beauty of their natural curls. Here's a list of the bloggers whose websites and YouTube channels I've visited and found helpful. You can also find most of them on Facebook.

- AfricanExport
- Afrobella.com
- Beautifulbrwnbabydol
- BlackGirlLongHair.com
- CharyJay
- Colored Beautiful.com
- CurlyNikki.com
- DPrincess28
- Going-natural.com
- Hairlista.com
- HairMilk.com
- Keep It Simple Sister (KISS)
- KimmayTube
- KinkyCoilyPamela
- LongHairCareForum.com
- KisForKinky.com
- Mahogany Curls.com
- MotownGirl.com

- MsVaughnTV
- Napnatural.com
- Nappturality.com
- NapturallyCurly.com
- Naturalhair.org
- Naturalhairbeauty.blogspot.com
- NaturallyCurly.com
- NaturallyLeslie.blogspot.com
- NaturalMe4c
- NewlyNatural.com
- Nikkimae2003
- PrettyDimples01
- QuestforthePerfectCurl (Elle)
- TarenGuy
- TheGoodHairBlog.com

For a more complete listing of blogs about natural hair, visit Networked Blogs at www.networkedblogs.com/topic/natural_hair.

Natural Hair Care Books

Part of your journey will be learning as much as possible about natural hair care. In addition to my sister bloggers, I also turned to books on natural hair. Today, there are several books to choose from and as the natural hair explosion expands, even more books will be hitting the market. I recommend that you check out the reader reviews on Amazon before purchasing.

This list is not exhaustive, but is a sampling of the natural hair books available at the time of publication of this resource guide.

- *10 Easy Steps To Go Natural Without Cutting Your Hair Off!* (Volume 1) by Nik Scott (2012).

- *10 Secrets to Growing Black Hair Long and Fast* by C. Collins (2013).

- *55 Fun & Fabulous DIY Beauty Recipes: Natural Homemade Skin, Hair, & Nail Care Recipes Using Aromatherapy Essential Oils (Holistic Tips, Recipes & Remedies Series)* by Amy Waldow (2013).

- *Afros: A Celebration of Natural Hair* by Michael July (2013).

- *Better Than Good Hair: The Curly Girl Guide to Healthy, Gorgeous Natural Hair!* by Nikki Walton and Ernessa T. Carter (2013).

- *Coif Cuisine: Natural Hair Recipes & Side Dishes for the Natural Hair and Now* by Candace O. Kelley (2011).

- *Coils & Curls The Hair Product Handbook: Helping the Product Junkies of the world buy SMARTER, sort through marketing HYPE and save MONEY!* by Nicole Harmon (2012).

- *Curly Girl: The Handbook* by Lorraine Massey (2011).

- *Curly Like Me: How to Grow Your Hair Healthy, Long and Strong* by Teri LaFlesh (2010).

- *Get Your Length! Helping Women with Natural Hair Retain Length* by Sais Sharpe and Anthony Policastro (2013).

- *Going-Natural: How to Fall in Love with Nappy Hair* by Mireille Liong-a-kong (2004).

- *Going Natural: How to Transition from Relaxed Hair to Natural Hair in 7 Simple Steps* by Jael Byrd and Kenneth Byrd (2011).

- *Good Hair* by Lonnice Brittenum Bonner (1990).

- *Good Hair: For Colored Girls Who've Considered Weaves When the Chemicals Became Too Ruff* by Lonnice Brittenum Bonner (1994).

- *Grow It: How to Grow Afro-Textured Hair to Maximum Lengths in the Shortest Time* by Chicoro (2008).

- *Grow it Kinky: How to Grow Long Kinky Natural Hair* by Ariane Roberts, Vanessa Roberts, Mike Dimock and Meghan Reid (2013).

- *Hair Care Rehab: The Ultimate Hair Repair & Reconditioning Manual* by Audrey Davis-Sivasothy (2012).

- *Hair Rules!: The Ultimate Hair-Care Guide for Women with Kinky, Curly, or Wavy Hair* Anthony Dickey (2003).

- *Hair Story: Untangling The Roots of Black Hair in America* by Ayana D. Byrd & Lori L. Tharps (2002).

- *How to Go Natural Without Going Broke* by Crystal Swain-Bates (2013).

- *How to Grow Black Natural Hair* by Jael Byrd and Kenneth Byrd (2012).

- *If You Love It, It Will Grow: A Guide to Healthy, Beautiful Natural Hair* by Phoenyx Austin (2012).

- *Let's Talk Hair: Every Black Woman's Personal Consultation for Healthy Growing Hair* by Pamela Ferrell (1996).

- *Milady Standard: Natural Hair Care and Braiding* by Diane Carol Bailey and Diane Da Costa (2013).

- *Nappturosity: How to Create Fabulous Natural Hair and Locs* by Erin Shell Anthony (2007).

- *Natural Beauty Tips of the Ancients: Learn the secrets of using common household items to reveal your natural beauty and radiance* by Kalilia Bina (2013).

- *Natural Hair Care: A Guide to Transition and Beyond* by Breena Jaye (2012).

- *Natural Care for Curls and Kinks* by Todra Payne (2012).

- *Natural Hair and Hair Products* by Denika Penn-Carothers (2012).

- *Natural Hair Care and Braiding* by Diane Carol Bailey (1997).

- *Natural Hair for Young Women* by Phylecia Tarael-ANU (Author), Aimè Tudor-ANU (Editor), H. Yuya Assaan-ANU (Editor) (2013).

- *Natural Hair Journey: The Best Way to Transition to Natural Hair* by Lea Brown (2012).

- *Natural Hair Revolution & Resolutions...Kinky Hair Stories* by René Michelle Floyt (2011).

- *Nice Dreads: Hair Care Basics and Inspiration for Colored Girls Who've Considered Locking Their Hair* by Lonnice Brittenum Bonner (2005).

- *Reclaim Natural Beauty: How to Grow, Nourish, and Strengthen Natural, Black Hair* by Camille A. Jefferson (2011).

- *Regrowing Hair Naturally: Effective Remedies and Natural Treatments for Men and Women with Alopecia Areata, Alopecia Androgenetica, Telogen Effluvium and Other Hair Loss Problems* by Vera Peiffer (2013).

- *Secrets Of A Long-Term Transitioner* by Kai Chic (2011).

- *Textured Tresses: The Ultimate Guide to Maintaining and Styling Natural Hair* by Diane Da Costa with Paula T. Renfroe (2004).

- *Thank God I'm Natural: The Ultimate Guide to Caring for and Maintaining Natural Hair* by Chris-Tia Donaldson (2009).

- *The Black Hair Care Revolution: A Simple Pocket Guide to Growing & Maintaining Healthy Natural & Permed Hair* by Yetunde Jude, Betsy Bearden and Robert M. Henry (2009).

- *The Black Woman's Guide to Beautiful Hair: A Positive Approach to Maintaining Any Hair Type and Style* by Lisa Akbari (2002).

- *The Book of Natural Hair Questions & Answers (from a Stylist Perspective)* by Yesenia Hernandez (2013).

- *The Kitchen Beautician: Natural Hair Care Recipes for Beautiful Healthy Hair* by Dezarae Henderson (2013).

- *The Knotty Truth: Managing Tightly Coiled Hair at Home DIY Survival Guide* by Michele George (2009).

- *The Natural Hair Bible: The 10 Commandments of Black Hair Care* by Breanna Rutter and Jared Rutter (2013).

- *The Natural Hair Handbook: Everything You Need to Know About Natural Hair* by Shawntay Jones (2012).

- *The Natural Hair Handbook: The Definitive Guide to Natural Hair* by Deneita Walker (2012).

- *The Root of the Matter: A Natural Hair Self-Help Guide* by Lori Lindsey and Kimbley Miller (2012).

- *The Secrets Of Going Natural: The Ultimate Guide To Loving Your Natural Hair* by Zenobia Jackson and Anthony Jackson (2011).

- *What Works, What Doesn't in Healthy Hair Care* by Marleyna A. (2013).

Hair Care Lines with Products for Natural Hair

I've provided below a list of companies with products designed for kinky-textured hair. Every day, more and more companies and products are hitting the market, so by no means is this list exhaustive. I encourage you to take some time to visit each of these websites (use that hour you've set aside to deep condition each week) and check out their products. With so many products available to choose from, it's indeed a great time to be natural!

III Sisters of Nature
3sistersofnature.com

4 Naturals
4naturals.com

As I Am
asiamnaturally.com

Beija Flor Naturals
beijaflornaturals.com

Beautiful Textures
beautifultextures.com

Blended Beauty
blendedbeauty.com

Carol's Daughter
carolsdaughter.com

Curls Goddess Curls
curls.biz

Curls Unleashed
curlsunleashed.com

Dark and Lovely Au Naturale
softsheen-carson.com

Design Essentials
designessentials.com

Dr. Miracles
drmiracles.com

Eden Body Works
edenbodyworks.com

Entwine Couture
entwinecouture.com

Essentious
essentious.com

Hydratherma Natural
healthyhairjourney.com

Jane Carter Solutions
JaneCartersolutions.com

Kinky Curly
kinky-curly.com

Luv Naturals
luvnaturals.com

Miss Jessie's
missjessies.com

Mixed Chicks
mixedchicks.net

Organic Root Stimulator
orshaircare.com

Qhemet Biologics
qhemetbiologics.com

Shea Moisture
sheamoisture.com

Sofn'free GroHealthy
mmproducts.com/sofn'freegrohealthy

Taliah Waajid Natural Hair Products
naturalhair.org

TGIN
thankgodimnatural.com

Tropical Roots
mytropicalroots.com

Tukka Naturals
tukkanaturals.com

Uncle Funky's Daughter
unclefunkysdaughter.com

REFERENCES

A myriad of books, articles, websites, YouTube bloggers and my own personal experiences guided me in
gathering the information contained in this book. The
following resources were particularly helpful.

- *The Science of Black Hair: A Comprehensive
  Guide to Textured Hair Care* by Audrey Davis-
  Sivasothy (2011).

- CurlyNikki.com.

- BlackGirlLongHair.com.

THANKS FOR YOUR SUPPORT!

Thank you for purchasing *Kinky Coily: A Natural Hair Resource Guide!* I sincerely hope it helps you on your natural hair journey. If you enjoyed the book, it would mean a lot to me if you would take a few minutes to rate it on Amazon. Even better, write a short blurb. Good reviews are crucial to the success of any book, so you'd be doing me a big favor by posting a review.

I would also be hugely honored if you would visit my website at www.pamelasamuelsyoung.com and join my mailing list. You can also friend me on Facebook and follow me on Twitter and Instagram.

As an independently published author, word of mouth buzz is crucial. So please tell your friends and family (and even a stranger or two) about *Kinky Coily: A Natural Hair Resource Guide* and be sure to check out the *Kinky Coily Natural Hair Journal* as well as my mystery books.

Thanks again for your support!

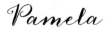

In addition to being a natural hair enthusiast,
Pamela Samuels Young is also an
award-winning mystery writer.
So be sure to check out her fast-paced thrillers.

To whet your appetite, here's a short excerpt from
one of her novels, which received an NAACP
Image Award for Outstanding Fiction.

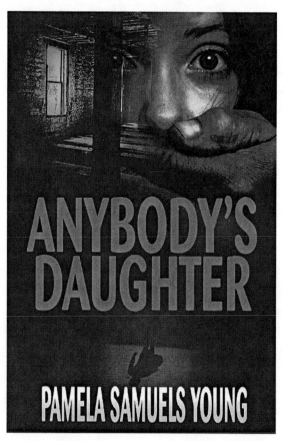

Prologue

BRIANNA SAT CROSS-LEGGED IN THE middle of her bed, her thumbs rhythmically tapping the screen of her iPhone. She paused, then hit the *Send* button, firing off the text message.

ready?

Soft hazel eyes lasered into the screen, anticipating—no craving—an instantaneous response. Jaden had told her to text him when she was about to leave the house. *So why didn't he respond?*

She hopped off the bed and cracked open the door. A gentle tinkle—probably a spoon clanking against the side of a stainless steel pot—signaled that her mother was busy in the kitchen preparing breakfast.

Easing the door shut, Brianna leaned against it and closed her eyes. She sucked in air through her nose and slowly released it through her lips, mimicking her mother in meditation. To pull this off, Brianna couldn't just act calm, she had to *be* calm. Otherwise, her mother would surely notice.

At thirteen, Brianna had no breasts to speak of, but she was quite proud of her small waist and her plump rear end, which was noticeably disproportionate to her otherwise-petite frame.

She gently shook the phone as if that might make Jaden's response instantly appear. Brianna was both thrilled and nervous about finally meeting Jaden, her first real boyfriend—a boyfriend she wasn't supposed to have. Texts and emails had been racing back and forth between them ever since Jaden friended her on Facebook five weeks earlier.

It still bothered Brianna—but only a little—that Jaden had refused to hook up with her on Skype or FaceTime or even talk to her on the phone. Jaden had explained that he wanted to hear her voice and see her face for the first time in person. When she thought about it, that *was* kind of romantic.

If it hadn't been for her Uncle Dre, Brianna would never have been able to have a secret boyfriend. When her uncle presented her with an iPhone for her birthday two months ago, her mother immediately launched into a tirade about perverts and predators on the Internet. But Uncle Dre had teased her mother for being so up-tight and successfully pleaded her case.

Thank God her mother was such a techno-square. Although she'd insisted that they share the same Gmail account and barred her from Facebook, Brianna simply used her iPhone to open a Facebook account using a Yahoo address that her mother knew nothing about. As for her texts, she immediately erased them.

A quiet chime signaled the message Brianna had been waiting for. A ripple of excitement shot through her.

Jaden: hey B almst there cant wait 2 c u.
Brianna: me 2
Jaden: cant wait 2 kss dem lips
Brianna: lol!
Jaden: luv u grl!
Brianna: luv u 2

Brianna tossed the phone onto the bed and covered her mouth with both hands.

OMG!

She was finally going to meet the love of her life. Jaden's older brother Clint was taking them to the Starbucks off Wilmington. Her mother kept such tight reins on her, this was the only time she could get away. Jaden had assured her that Clint would make sure she got to school on time.

Turning around to face the mirror on the door, Brianna untied her bushy ponytail and let her hair fall across her shoulders. The yellow-and-purple Lakers tank top her Uncle Dre had given her fit snugly across her chest, but wasn't slutty-looking. Jaden was a Kobe Bryant fanatic just like she was. He would be impressed when she showed up sporting No. 24.

Brianna slung her backpack over her shoulder and trudged down the hallway toward the kitchen.

"Hey, Mama. I have to be at school early for a Math Club meeting."

Donna Walker turned away from the stove. "I'm making pancakes. You don't have time for breakfast?"

Brianna felt a stab of guilt. Her mother was trying harder than ever to be a model parent. Brianna had spent much of the last year living with her grandmother after her mother's last breakdown.

"Sorry." She grabbed a cinnamon-raisin bagel from the breadbox on the counter. "Gotta go."

Donna wiped her hand on a dishtowel. "It's too early for you to be walking by yourself. I can drop you off."

Brianna's breath caught, but she kept her face neutral. "No need. I'm picking up Sydney. We're walking together."

Brianna saw the hesitation in her mother's overprotective eyes.

Taller and darker than her daughter, Donna wore her hair in short, natural curls. Her lips came together like two plump pillows and her eyes were a permanently sad shade of brown.

Donna had spent several years as a social worker, but now worked as an administrative assistant at St. Francis Hospital. Work, church and Brianna. That was her mother's entire life. No man, no girlfriends, no fun.

Brianna wasn't having any of that. She was *gonna* have a life, no matter how hard her mother tried to keep her on a short leash like a prized pet.

Donna finally walked over and gave her daughter a peck on the cheek, then repeated the same words she said every single morning: "You be careful."

Brianna bolted through the front door and hurried down the street. As expected, no one was out yet. Her legs grew shaky as she scurried past Sydney's house.

Brianna had wanted to tell her BFF about hooking up with Jaden today, but he made her promise not to. Anyway, Sydney had the biggest mouth in the whole seventh grade. Brianna couldn't afford to have her business in the street. She'd made Sydney swear on the Bible before telling her about Jaden.

As she neared the end of the block, she saw it. The burgundy Escalade with the tinted windows was parked behind Mario's Fish Market just like Jaden had promised. Brianna was so excited her hands began to tremble. She was only a few feet away from the SUV when the driver's door opened and a man climbed out.

"Hey, Brianna. I'm Clint, Jaden's brother. He's in the backseat."

Brianna unconsciously took a step back. Jaden's brother didn't look anything like him. On his Facebook picture, Jaden had dark eyes, a narrow nose and could've passed for T.I.'s twin brother. This man was dark-skinned with a flat nose and crooked teeth. And there was no way he was nineteen. He had to be even older than her Uncle Dre, who was thirty-something.

Brianna bit her lip. Something unsettling tinkered in her gut, causing her senses to see-saw between fear and elation. But it was love, her love for Jaden, that won out. It didn't matter what his brother looked like. They probably had different daddies.

She handed Clint her backpack and stooped to peer inside the back of the SUV.

At the same horrifying moment that Brianna realized that the man inside was not Jaden, Clint snatched her legs out from under her and shoved her inside the Escalade.

The man in the backseat grabbed a handful of her hair and jerked her toward him. Brianna tumbled face-first into his lap, inhaling sweat and weed and piss.

"Owwwww! Get your hands offa me!" Brianna shouted, her arms and legs thrashing about like a drowning swimmer. "Where's Jaden? Let me go!"

"Relax, baby." The stinky man's voice sounded old and husky. "Just calm down."

"Let me go!" Brianna screamed.

She tried to pull away, but Stinky Man palmed the back of her head like a basketball, easily holding her in place. Clint reached between the front seats, snatched her arms behind her back and bound them with rope.

When Brianna heard the quiet revving of the engine and the door locks click into place, panic exploded from her ears. She violently kicked her feet, hoping to break the window. But each kick landed with a sharp thud that fired needles of pain back up her legs.

"Don't touch me! Let me goooooo!"

The stinky man thrust a calloused hand down the back of her pants.

"Damn, girl," he cackled. "I like this big old ghetto booty."

"Cut it out, Leon," Clint shouted. "I've told you before. Don't mess with the merchandise."

Clint reached into the backseat again and stabbed Brianna's arm with a needle just above the elbow.

A flash of fire lit up her entire body and in seconds, her eyelids felt like two heavy windows being forced shut. She tried to scream, but the ringing in her ears drowned out all sound. When she blinked up at Stinky Man, he had two—no three—heads.

Brianna could feel the motion of the SUV pulling away from Mario's Fish Market. She needed to do something. But her body was growing heavy and her head ached. The thick haze that cluttered her mind allowed only one desperate thought to seep through.

Mommy! Uncle Dre! Please help me!

Anybody's Daughter and all of Pamela's novels are available in print, e-book and audio book formats, everywhere books are sold. To read an excerpt of Pamela's books, visit www.pamelasamuelsyoung.com.

BOOKS BY
PAMELA SAMUELS YOUNG

Vernetta Henderson Mysteries

Every Reasonable Doubt (1st in series)

In Firm Pursuit (2nd in series)

Murder on the Down Low (3rd in series)

Attorney-Client Privilege (4th in series)

Angela Evans Mysteries

Buying Time (1st in series)

Anybody's Daughter (2nd in series)

Short Stories

The Setup

Easy Money

Non-Fiction

Kinky Coily: A Natural Hair Resource Guide

Kinky Coily Natural Hair Journal

ABOUT THE AUTHOR

Pamela Samuels Young is a practicing attorney and award-winning author of the legal thrillers, *Every Reasonable Doubt, In Firm Pursuit, Murder on the Down Low, Buying Time, Attorney-Client Privilege,* and *Anybody's Daughter.* She is also a natural hair enthusiast and the author of K*inky Coily: A Natural Hair Resource Guide* and the *Kinky Coily Natural Hair Journal.*

In addition to writing legal thrillers and working as an in-house employment attorney for a major corporation in Southern California, Pamela formerly served on the board of directors of the Los Angeles Chapter of Mystery Writers of America and is a diehard member of Sisters in Crime-L.A., an organization dedicated to the advancement of women mystery writers. The former journalist and Compton native is a graduate of USC, Northwestern University and UC Berkeley's School of Law. She is single and lives in the Los Angeles area.

Pamela loves to hear from readers! There are a multitude of ways to connect with her.

Facebook

www.facebook.com/pamelasamuelsyoung

www.facebook.com/kinkycoilypamela

Twitter

www.twitter.com/pamsamuelsyoung

LinkedIn

www.linkedin.com/pamelasamuelsyoung

Pinterest

www.pinterest.com/kinkycoily

Instagram

www.instagram/pamelasamuelsyoung

YouTube

www.youtube.com/kinkycoilypamela.

MeetUp

www.meetup.com/natural-born-beauties

To schedule Pamela for a speaking engagement, conference or a book club meeting via speakerphone, Skype, FaceTime or in person, visit her website at www.pamelasamuelsyoung.com.

CPSIA information can be obtained at www.ICGtesting.com
Printed in the USA
LVOW06s0102251115

464121LV00001B/15/P